The Children in

Rutgers Series in Childhood Studies

The Rutgers Series in Childhood Studies is dedicated to increasing our understanding of children and childhoods throughout the world, reflecting a perspective that highlights cultural dimensions of the human experience. The books in this series are intended for students, scholars, practitioners, and those who formulate policies that affect children's everyday lives and futures.

Series Board

For a list of all the titles in the series, please see the last page of the book.

The Children in Child Health

Negotiating Young Lives and Health in New Zealand

JULIE SPRAY

RUTGERS UNIVERSITY PRESS

NEW BRUNSWICK, CAMDEN, AND NEWARK, NEW JERSEY, AND LONDON

LIBRARY OF CONGRESS CATALOGING-IN-PUBLICATION DATA

Names: Spray, Julie, author.
Title: The children in child health: negotiating young lives and health
in New Zealand / Julie Spray.
Description: New Brunswick: Rutgers University Press, [2020] | Series: Rutgers series
in childhood studies | Includes bibliographical references and index.
Identifiers: LCCN 2019019229 | | ISBN 9781978809314 (cloth) ISBN 9781978809307 (pbk.)
Subjects: LCSH: Children—Health and hygiene—New Zealand. |
Children—Social aspects—New Zealand.
Classification: LCC RJ103.N45 S67 2020 | DDC 362.19892000993—dc23
LC record available at https://lccn.loc.gov/2019019229

A British Cataloging-in-Publication record for this book is
available from the British Library.

www.rutgersuniversitypress.org

Manufactured in the United States of America

For the children of Aotearoa

Ahakoa he iti, he pounamu.
Although small, it is valuable.
—Māori proverb

CONTENTS

The Children in Child Health

1

Introduction

Nine-year-old Victor[1] "cannot tell a lie," his mother Adrienne tells me. The youngest of four boys, he would go out with his brothers, who would warn him, "Don't tell Mum that we went for a *kai* [feed]." Back home, Adrienne would ask whether he enjoyed his time. "Yup," Victor would reply. "I didn't go to McDonald's."

"Oh, you went to McDonald's, aye?!"

"No, I didn't!" Victor would protest. "I didn't have a cheeseburger!"

Victor's honesty, which could embarrass his mother and frequently got him into trouble at school, was much more useful to me as a researcher. Making lists at his kitchen table about "what it means to be a child" and "what it means to be an adult," Victor's mother puts her head in her hands as he explains to me that "adults don't have enough money, so you got to drip-dry your towels"; that adults have to put their cold food in the cupboard rather than a refrigerator; and that adults "need money to afford a lighter, or you can't buy your packets of smokes."[2]

It seems that Victor's experience of adults is seeing them struggle. His ideas about childhood and adulthood are shaped by the material deprivation of his family, in turn a product of national and global political, economic and historical forces. A history of colonialism and neoliberal economic policy in Aotearoa,[3] or New Zealand, has widened inequality and exacerbated a housing crisis within the Auckland region, both of which disproportionately affect Māori families like Victor's, as well as the families of many of his Pasifika[4] classmates (Amore 2016). For those growing up in poverty, these conditions of inadequate housing, nutrition, and health care in turn create a particular experience of childhood. As this book will show, how children interpret the circumstances of their childhoods matters, not least because these understandings shape children's practices: the way they negotiate their relationships, the way they approach risk, and the way

1

they manage their bodies. While the political and economic forces of society shape children's health from above, this is not the whole story; children's interpretations of and responses to their experiences further mediate these effects. Child health is therefore a coproduction, and a full understanding of the dynamics of child health requires both a view of the broader workings of society and a view from children's eyes, as experienced from within a child's body.

Victor's experience of childhood, like that of many other children I worked with, is one of chronic ill health originating from the quicksand of poverty. When Victor was four, Adrienne moved into a three-bedroom house owned by an acquaintance. The family soon discovered the house was in poor condition. "We were in a house that kind of lifted up a bit off the ground," Adrienne explains, "and underneath the house was full of water. It was full of water, and it wasn't insulated—"

"There was holes in the roof," Victor interjects.

Six months after they moved in, five-year-old Victor was hospitalized with heart valve damage following rheumatic fever.

From Adrienne's perspective, the poor housing conditions were to blame for Victor's illness. He was healthy before they moved. Adrienne tried asking the landlord for heating and finally tried taking the case to court, without success. With a poor credit rating and supporting four children on a single income, Adrienne found herself trapped; while she had a roof over her head, Housing New Zealand would not assess her for state housing,[5] but her landlord would not make the improvements she needed. The family remained in the house for another four and a half years, while Adrienne researched the causes of rheumatic fever and worked to combat the dampness that the landlord would not address. But the house was sitting atop about four inches of water, while the surrounding grass would sink after rain to form a pool so deep "you could have like a swim there." Adrienne scrubbed the mildew-riddled rooms every week so that her children could breathe.

After five years, the rent was raised so high that Adrienne could no longer afford to pay. The family moved in with Adrienne's sister—where I first visited them—and applied to Housing New Zealand (the state housing provider) for assistance. Because of Victor's heart condition, the family's application was prioritized, and when I visited them again three months later, they had relocated to a state house in the same area. Adrienne was delighted with her new home: insulated, clean, and dry.

Yet Victor's body will always bear the marks of the conditions of his early life, and this is the body through which he experiences his childhood. At nine years old, he understands his heart has been damaged and he cannot play rugby like his brothers and classmates, or go on the Fearfall ride at the local theme park. Between his heart condition and his asthma, Victor struggles to move physically, and as a consequence of this difficulty, along with poor nutrition, he is obese. His large size has likely contributed to his sleep apnea, which keeps him awake at night, as do his eczema and, even more so, his coughing from asthma. He sleepwalks, and his mother often finds him in front of the television in the wee hours of the morning when he can't sleep. His skin is riddled with rashes, pockmarks, and small sores; his nose runs from hay fever; and he is prone to nosebleeds. Some of these conditions may improve, but his life has to some degree been set on a trajectory of poor health and social stigma.

How Do Children Participate in the Coproduction of Their Health?

Victor's heart condition is currently managed under the District Health Board (DHB)[6] with monthly prophylactic penicillin injections, administered at his school by a visiting public health nurse. Victor is not a passive recipient of care, however, but responds with his own set of practices born of his social environment, including at school. When he is called to the office to get his injection, he tells his class he is in trouble, reinforcing his identity as social deviant. He steals packets of cookies from Adrienne's cupboard to take to school for lunch, which, whether he so intends or not, inevitably end up shared among the children in his class. On one day, unable to swallow the antibiotics administered by the school clinic for a strep throat, he covertly spat his pills into the rubbish bin, covered them with paper, thanked the nurse, and returned to class. His health, therefore, is a product not only of what is done to him, but also of how he makes sense of and negotiates a body lived within a social world he himself helps to create.

The way that children understand and respond to illness and its treatment therefore can have significant impact on how policies play out and what consequences they might have. The structural determinants of child health in Aotearoa have been extensively discussed in health and social science literature. They also are, to some extent, addressed in public health policy and services, which, for example, provide subsidized insulation to improve housing and targeted funding for community services (e.g., Telfar-Barnard, Preval, Howden-Chapman, et al. 2011). While the roles of the state, medical professionals, schools, and parents are accounted for within child health policy, the roles children themselves play in their own health care tend to remain invisible. With a view of children as passive, lacking competency, and vulnerable, the public policy approach since the landmark 1989 Children, Young Persons, and Their Families Act[7] has increasingly been oriented toward protecting children by regulating their lives (Tap 2007) within a social investment paradigm concerned with maximizing human capital and minimizing future expense (Elizabeth and Larner 2009; Keddell 2018; O'Brien 2016). This assumption of adult control over children's lives may underlie the lack of attention paid to children's experience of health policy and of their bodies themselves. But what happens to children's experience of their bodies when they are asked every day to check on an aspect of their health? How do children come to define "lunch" when governments say that good parents provide them with meals they do not have? What happens to children's health care practices when illness is discursively linked to death?

These are questions not only about individual behavior, but also about how broader structural conditions (institutional, socioeconomic, political, demographic) are experienced through bodies and translated into social meanings and practices within children's peer cultures. I argue that the answers to these questions *matter* because the social meanings children produce from their structured, embodied experience in turn reinforce, modify, or generate biosocial practices of the body.

I use the term "coproduction" to characterize these processes, though what I mean by the term varies slightly from other scholars' use of the concept. From a Science, Technology and Society (STS) perspective, Sheila Jasanoff (2004) refers to the mutually constituting nature of science and society, whereby social, legal, and political institutions both shape and are shaped by scientific knowledge and associated technologies. Here, the coproduction framework powerfully reveals how science, while purporting objectivity, becomes imbued with the biases and political motives of the humans who create science, as well as how, in part because of this presumed objectivity, science and technology can modify or legitimize the institutions, power structures, and values of society. Meanwhile, Margaret Lock (2001) writes of the coproduction between biology and culture that creates embodied experience. She points out that even the most basic of biological events are contingent on the interaction of individual biology with language; cultural understandings and categories of the body; and the organization of societies by class, age, gender, ethnicity, political-economic contexts, and diet or physical environment. Consequently, most experiences of the body—pain, hunger, illness—are variable, though when features of the sociocultural or physical environment are more or less shared, then individuals may also share aspects of their embodied experience. From these shared experiences of the body, people collectively generate cultural understandings and discourses of health, illness, development, aging, and suffering that in turn filter bodily experience. In this perspective, coproduction is constituted through the dialectic interaction of biology and culture, which sediment into what Lock terms "local biologies" of bodily experience.

Both authors, therefore, use coproduction to describe the dialectical nature of relationships—for Jasanoff, between science and society, and for Lock, between the body and culture. In this book, I employ a similar idea of coproduction to capture the way that children's health is produced through dialectical relationships among society, the body, and children's own practices. Importantly, the notion of coproduction offers a way of giving attention to children's activities as significant and powerful without implying that children are responsible for their own well-being. Victor's practices contribute to his health: lying to his class allows him to obtain the injections that prevent secondary rheumatic fever recurrence while avoiding the stress of stigma; stealing and sharing food shapes his nutritional status; spitting out his antibiotics alters the microbiology of his body. Yet all of these practices are also structured by Victor's body, the peer society he co-creates, and the wider social organization of the institution, the community, and the state. He lies to his class in part because of a health system that delivers care through the institution. He shares his cookies because of a peer culture that demands distribution of resources in a context of scarcity. He spits out his antibiotics because the pills are big for small throats and difficult to swallow, and because the alternative liquid medicine is socially understood to mark a "little kid." Finally, his practices also contribute to meanings within peer cultures—stigma, morality, identity—that maintain, reinforce, or transform the social structures that guide his activities as well as those of his peers, teachers, parents, and even policy makers. Coproduction therefore characterizes the way that children's health is made through collaboration between children and society: through practices that are both enacted through bodies and embodied, and that are structured by society just as they structure future action. What, then, are the processes through which children coproduce their own health and the health of others around them?

From Asthma to Rheumatic Fever

To answer this question, I spent a year, including holidays, driving more than an hour to the opposite side of the city to attend Tūrama School in Papakura, South Auckland. Almost every day, I worked alongside children aged between eight and twelve years (school years five through eight)[8] to research their understandings and experiences of health and illness. As a place where the state directly reaches children's lives in significant ways, a school setting offered the opportunity to observe how children's peer cultures interact with government policy to coproduce health.

I was introduced to Tūrama School by a former work colleague, Mrs. Randall, who was now a senior teacher there. On my behalf, she asked the principal whether I could conduct my research with the school while acting as an informal teacher aide. After meeting with the principal and gaining ethics approval, in 2015 I eventually joined Mrs. Randall in her classroom where I was based for the first few months of fieldwork, building a solid set of relationships with the twenty-two children there. After a while, I began to visit six other classes, initially rotating day by day, and later focusing on sustained work with just three, though I still visited the others regularly. I volunteered my services as a "classroom helper," an offer which some teachers took up more than others. I mounted work, cut up labels, taught art lessons, and accompanied classes on myriad field trips:

athletics day, swimming sports day, the museum, the local theme park, end-of-year trips for the graduating year sixes. I also filled two workbooks with handwriting and mathematics exercises, spelling words and diagrams of volca-noes, as I worked alongside children in the classroom, moving around different groups of children as I usually took the spare desk of whoever was away that day.

My original plan was to focus on asthma, a disease that is very common among New Zealand children and disproportionately affects Māori and Pasifika children (Ellison-Loschmann, Pattemore, Asher, et al. 2009). I proposed to estab-lish myself within a school, observing how asthma plays out within a context of everyday health meanings and practices at school, while also inviting children with asthma and their families to participate in a focused asthma study across the year at home. I introduced myself to each class as an anthropologist, retell-ing "the story of Myra"—Myra Bluebond-Langner's (1978) famous study of dying children—as a way of illustrating how adults don't always know things about children, and how children and anthropologists together can help adults to understand children better. ("Now you are not dying," I would hasten to add. "But I think there are important things about your lives that adults *think* they know about, but they don't really. Do you?") This introduction was part of an ethical mode of research that aimed for transparency and partnership as much as pos-sible, in order to create safety and trust, and to model respect for *children's* boundaries as much as I expected them to respect mine. Any interested child took home an information pack, and out of approximately 150 students, fifty-three girls and twenty-eight boys returned both signed child assent forms and adult consent forms granting me permission to write notes about the child at the end of each school day. In my contact and relationships with the children during school, I made no differentiation between those who had consented and those who had not.

Though I was able to recruit eighty-one children for the school study, and seven children into the asthma study, it became apparent within the first few months that though asthma was common, it was not particularly salient among the complex of intersecting threats to well-being and the complicated sets of practices children and parents used to negotiate these. When children are expe-riencing the demands of poor nutrition, cold, stress, infections, insufficient sleep, bullying, domestic violence, addiction, family illness, and social instabil-ity, to focus on asthma seemed rather like missing the forest for the trees. More-over, high rates of rheumatic fever among this group of children meant that Tūrama School, like other schools in low-income communities, was the target of a government program that included a public health promotion campaign and a school-based clinic. These interventions were powerful intrusions into school life and begged for attention to children's perspectives that had until then been neglected in policy. While I continued working with the families in the asthma study, I initiated a third component to the research, inviting all children, with or without their families as they wished, to participate in an open-ended interview about health and illness more generally, and strep throat and rheumatic fever in particular. An additional thirty-eight children participated, some in pairs or threes, and several, having enjoyed the experience, participated in a second interview. I also interviewed four teachers, the deputy principal, the school social worker, the clinic nurse, and six parents or caregivers, as well as formally or informally meeting an assortment of other *whānau*[9] (family) members.

How Are Children Actors in Their Health Care?

In writing about New Zealand children, I follow a long legacy of anthropologists researching childhoods and families in the Pacific. This legacy includes significant ethnographic work on child-rearing in Aotearoa and Polynesia by Waikato psychologists Jane and James Ritchie, whose publications span almost half a century (examples include Ritchie 1957; Ritchie and Ritchie 1970, 1979, 1997). Throughout this work, the Ritchies argue strongly for a distinct pattern of Māori child-rearing, based on evidence collected over time and space, and are vocal advocates for this pattern to be recognized in policy and social services, and for child and Māori rights more generally. Joan Metge also pays attention to Māori children as positioned within the whānau (Metge 1967, 1995). More recently, Relinde Tap writes of Pākehā (New Zealand European) and Dutch childhoods from the perspective of parents (Tap 2007), and a body of anthropological work on children has appeared in relation to health, again mainly from the perspective of parents (Mavoa 2004; Park 2000; Scott, Laing, and Park 2016; Trnka 2017). Across the Pacific, anthropologists have conducted ethnographic work on children and families, particularly debating questions of how children become acculturated adults and how families distribute child-rearing, for example in Samoa (Holmes 1974; Mead 1930), Tonga (Morton 1996), and Fiji (Toren 1990; also Karen Brison's [2014] work on identities). Given the strong focus on socialization however, children's own experiences, perspectives, and cultures have been the subject of less anthropological attention in this part of the world (though Mead [1930] and Morton [1996] both interviewed adolescents), and to my knowledge, this book represents the first substantive ethnographic representation of children's own cultural production in a Pacific context.

I therefore find my analysis of children's cultural production and health situates itself within the interpretive childhood literature, in which the significance of children's meaning-making to health is well represented by a stream of child-centered studies of illness, largely based in western Europe or North America (Bluebond-Langner 2000, 1978; Christensen 1999; Clark 2003; James 1993; Mayall 1996; Prout 1986, 2000a; Prout and Christensen 1996; but also see Hunleth 2017, in Zambia). Beginning with Myra Bluebond-Langner's (1978) ethnography of children with terminal cancer, interest in children's illness perspectives burgeoned at the end of the twentieth century following the emer-gence of what is sometimes termed the new social studies of childhood (NSSC) and James and Prout's (1990) call to view childhood as a culturally constructed product of a given society. Central to these studies is the recognition of children's agency: their capacity to produce their own meanings and practices in relation to illness, which are distinct from, but influenced by, adult notions and prac-tices. For example, in an ethnography of children's chronic illness, Cindy Dell Clark (2003) illustrates the many creative ways that children use "imaginal cop-ing" to transform the discomforts and mundanities of diabetes or asthma into fantasy, play, humor, or ritual. Children can also demonstrate their agency by manipulating adult constructs of illness. In a study of a small English commu-nity, Alan Prout (1986) showed how children could work with social meanings of illness to influence adults' decision-making—for example, by feigning or dis-guising symptoms.

This movement toward recognizing children as social actors has therefore been an important reconfiguring of assumptions about children's role in their health care. However, while numerous analyses consider how children's bodies may affect their experiences and meaning-making, the interpretive literature on child health generally stops short of analyzing how children's practices may impact their biology. Yet asking how children contribute to their bodies reveals the limitations of agency as an analytical concept in the face of another prob-lem: how to position children as social actors without implying responsibility for well-being.

Indeed, a number of scholars have cautioned against using agency too uncritically in analyses of childhood (Ansell 2014; Campbell, Andersen, Mutsikiwa, et al. 2015; Durham 2008; Lancy 2012; Mizen and Ofosu-Kusi 2013). Interpretive studies of childhood can tend toward a romanticized depiction of resilient and resourceful children making creative choices to overcome adver-sity, while masking the constraints on their choices, the extent of their suffer-ing, and the conditions under which children do not have agency (Prout 2000a). Campbell and colleagues argue against this tendency to view agency as a child's ability to engage in any form of action per se, referencing Andersen's (2012) point that agency is "a blunt analytical tool to describe a 12-year-old girl's choice to have unprotected sex with an HIV-positive older man, to generate income to feed her younger siblings" (cf. Campbell, Andersen, Mutsikiwa, et al. 2015, 55).

Yet studies of how children's health is produced have tended to avoid the issue of how children use agency, pointing upstream to the historical, social, and political-economic factors and cultural ideologies that structure people's lives and practices. The power of global political, economic, and social forces to shape childhoods has been well recognized in anthropology (Scheper-Hughes 1996; Stephens 1995). Critical studies of childhood, like Kristen Cheney's (2017) analysis of children orphaned by the HIV/AIDS epidemic in Uganda, consider the impact of inequality, from the local scale to the global. A body of research in biological anthropology considers the impact of policies and structures on children's bodies; biological outcomes such as physical growth or morbidity rates are employed to measure the effects of disparities in exposure to risk or access to care and material resources (Bogin and Loucky 1997; Panter-Brick 1998b). However, in this literature children tend to be positioned as passive experiencers and absorbers of the conditions that impact them. In his chapter on childhoods in the crack houses of East Harlem, for example, Philippe Bourgois (1995, 261) powerfully describes the children he encounters as becoming "ground up" into the underclass as they internalize the conditions of the barrio. Yet as those interpretive studies of childhood agency have demonstrated so emphatically, children are also engaged in the production of culture, so the concept of internalization is not sufficient to explain the processes of social reproduction. How, then, to position children as contributors to health when much of their health status is, like Victor's, the product of powerfully converging historical, social, and political economic forces?

To resolve this question, I draw on the theoretical work of sociologists William Corsaro (1992, 2015), Pierre Bourdieu (1977, 1984), Chris Shilling (1993), and Alan Prout (2000b, 2005) to unravel the way children's practices contribute to the coproduction of their health through their engagement with and transformation of the social structures that guide and constrain children's practices. These scholars all deal with issues of structure, agency, and the body in social reproduction. While Bourdieu is more focused on the structures and outcomes of socialization in the form of the internalized "habitus," Corsaro does the work of isolating the mechanisms of socialization and expanding these beyond internalization to children's cultural appropriation, reinvention, and reproduction. However, Bourdieu's conception of embodied practices constructing and constructed by social structures brings a necessary view of the way children's interpretive practices are constrained and guided by the circumstances within which these practices are produced. Shilling, also drawing from Bourdieu, elaborates on how these practices articulate with biological bodies, and Prout extends Shilling's biosocial theory to children, laying the foundations for understanding the dynamics of children's participation in the coproduction of their health. Though they may not use the term "coproduction," all of these scholars are concerned with how individuals—or individual bodies—and society produce one another, and thus their insights contribute to my analysis of how children, together with society, come to coproduce their health.

Each of these theorists emerge from concurrent, distinct, though interconnected lineages of twentieth century scholarship across anthropology, sociology, and psychology. In the remainder of this chapter I therefore trace the ways that questions of children and social reproduction have been dealt with through parallel lines of inquiry through socialization, practice theory, and developmental psychology. In particular, I note four major shifts in thinking about childhood that lay the groundwork for this book: first, the movement toward recognizing children's agency within their socialization; second, the understanding of agency as working dialectically with structure; third, the extension of socialization processes beyond individual internalization to a collective and transformative reproduction; and finally a view of the body as biosocially produced.

Finding Agency in Socialization

The term "socialization" is used to describe the processes through which individuals—particularly children—become members of society and society reproduces itself. Interest in these processes developed across the social and psychological sciences of the early twentieth-century United States, where the decline of child mortality as a result of public health measures and mass enrollment in secondary schooling generated new attention to childhood in what LeVine (2007) calls "pediatric and pedagogical terms" (248). In psychology, this meant the emergence of modern developmental psychology, which sought to understand the cognitive and socioemotional processes through which children grow into adults. For anthropology, the subsequent wave of psychological theory around the child, including the theories of Freud, Piaget, Vygotsky, and Bowlby, generated much of the agenda in the United States, and a proliferation of child-rearing and cultural transmission studies documented the variation in socialization practices and effects across cultures (Montgomery 2009). These studies included the influential Culture and Personality studies led by pioneering anthropologists such as Ruth Benedict, Margaret Mead, and Edward Sapir, which set out to address empirical questions about the relationship between childhood experiences and enculturated adults (Schwartzman 2001). In general, these studies and those that have followed are concerned with the ways in which adults mold children into particular kinds of social citizens; the child here is mostly passive but embedded in social relations and interactions.

To this day, anthropologists remain interested in the processes of socialization (Bolin 2006; Briggs 1970, 1979; Broch 1990; Geurts 2003; Morton 1996; Chapin 2014). However, the literature has evolved, in part under the influence of the new childhood studies in the early 1990s, which emphasized children's agency and expanded consideration of socializing agents from the parent to the wider family, including children themselves, the community, and peer group. For example, Brigg's (1998) study of Inuit socialization follows a single three-year-old child, positioning her as an active agent in every interaction documented and inferring her perspectives where possible. Such a reconsideration of children's agency in socialization processes also emerged from the language socialization subfield of linguistics, which criticized traditional anthropological socialization for treating children as the passive recipients of culture and over-looking how everyday language functions as a key medium of socialization. Instead, scholars working from a language socialization paradigm examine how the processes of linguistic and cultural development are interlinked, and these scholars highlight the active role of the child in acquiring *and* generating language (Heath 1983; Ochs 1993; Schieffelin 1990; Schieffelin and Ochs 1986). Meanwhile, some branches of childhood anthropology, such as studies of cognition and learning, have moved away from socialization frameworks, instead following the developmental psychology of Piaget and Vygotsky to center the child as the agent acquiring the understanding. For example, Christina Toren (1993, 1999) explicitly rejects socialization as something adults do to children, instead arguing that although others help create the structures, it is the individual who constitutes their own meanings from these structures, in a process she calls human autopoiesis, or self-making.

More recently, Allison James presents an extensive "child-centered" study of socialization from children's own perspectives using Smart's (2007) frame of the personal life (James 2013). Asking what socialization from a child's perspective would look like, James bridges the large gap between the decades-long concern with child-rearing for social reproduction and the NSSC's preoccupation with agency. She explores how children experience, perceive, negotiate, and transform various traditional institutions of socialization—the family, the school—in collective and embodied ways. This creates a shift from seeing families and institutions as socializing children to seeing how, through their involvement in the practices of these groups, children become socialized. As James engages in detail with practice theory, this work also represents a shift from the original childhood studies to consider when and how children's agency is subject to constraint. This version of children's agency is contingent and negotiated, working dialectically with the structures of the family, institutions, and society, coproducing *childhood*.

Theorizing Socialization and Social Reproduction

While the anthropologists of the mid-twentieth century tested psychological theories with ethnographic accounts of child-rearing across cultures, within this literary milieu sociologists also developed influential theories of socialization and social reproduction. Perhaps most significant of the early theorists is Talcott Parsons (1951), who drew on Durkheim to answer the Hobbesian problem of how order is maintained in society. For Parsons, the notion that social systems were entirely maintained through rules and laws was insufficient, as he noted that individuals tend to work in ways that sustain rather than destabilize systems (James 2013). Society does not simply impose social rules, Parsons argues;

instead, families and schools play a functional role in transmitting culture and practices to the next generation whereby, from a young age, children internalize social norms to the point that these norms become *self*-imposed.

Among other issues, it is this uninterrogated internalization concept that Dennis Wrong (1961) particularly critiques in what he labels an "oversocialised view of man" (184). Wrong argues that Parsons has misconstrued the original Freudian meaning of the term "internalization" to loosely mean "learning" or "habits," with the implication that the individual affirms as well as conforms to those norms. This interpretation neglects the "inner conflict" aspect of Freud's superego, which suggests only that an individual will feel guilty for not living up to a norm—not that the individual actually will conform. Internalization, as Parson uses the concept, is therefore an assumption of fact that is taken for granted and that, without an unpacking of the underlying mechanics, has limited explanatory power. In fact, Parson is simply reversing the question, Wrong points out, writing, "How is it that violence, conflict, revolution, and the individual's sense of coercion by society manage to exist at all, if this view is correct?" (186). What are the circumstances under which such "internalization" does not, or does not fully, occur?

Such opposition to the Parsonian view of individuals internalizing the rules of society, as well as the constraint-based theory of scholars concerned with hegemonies of power (Karl Marx, for instance), cognitive structures (Claude Levi-Strauss), or cultural systems (Clifford Geertz), gave rise to the practice theory of the 1970s and 1980s and its attempts to explain the relationships between human action and "the system" (Crossley 2001; Ortner 1984). Practice theorists such as Bourdieu (1977), Giddens (1979), and Sahlins (1981) argued for a dialectical rather than oppositional relationship between agentive practice and constraint; while social structures and systems constrain actors, the same structures and systems are also produced, reproduced, and can be transformed through practice—what people *do* (Miller and Goodnow 1995; Ortner 2006).

I focus here on Bourdieu in no small part because the embodied nature of habitus has important implications for the present study of health. Bourdieu's theory of practice involves individuals as social actors deploying different forms of "capital" (economic, social, or symbolic assets) in strategic negotiations across different "fields," or distinct domains of action, such as home, work, and school (Bourdieu 1977, 1986). Central is Bourdieu's concept of "habitus," an enduring and transferable set of schemes internalized within individuals through the repetitious practice of certain modes of being, thinking, and behaving, which sediment into largely unconscious, predisposing structures for future action (Wacquant 2005; Maton 2008). In other words, people become what they do and do what they become. What people do, however, is also guided by pre-existing historical, social, and environmental structures such as class and material opportunities that constrain possible actions or that constrain *perceptions* of

possible actions. For example, Connolly (2004) describes how children who succeed in school tend to come from middle-class homes where they have acquired
the "dispositions" and educational capital from parents who themselves value
and encourage engagement in education and possess the forms of knowledge
hegemonic in the national curriculum. These processes explain the tendencies of gender or class structures to reproduce themselves, as individuals experiencing common conditions (and *conditionings*) will share characteristics of the
habitus but also perceive these commonalities to reflect the natural or com-
monsense order of things (doxa) (Bourdieu 1977). Yet while Bourdieu's habitus
has, at times, been criticized for being overly deterministic in that individuals
are born into a structured world that predates them (Jenkins 1982), Bourdieu
conceptualizes these matrices as circular and evolving; the structured world has
been constructed by prior individuals, and will form a base from which future
individuals will reproduce, innovate, and generate new structures that predispose rather than predetermine future action (Crossley 2001).

Childhood is a period of critical importance for Bourdieu because within
early childhood the primary habitus is laid down, setting the trajectory for
(though not wholly determining) an individual's lifelong embodied practice
(Bourdieu 1984). In recognizing the "structuring activity of agents" (467), Bourdieu
leaves open the possibility that children too could be agents who engage in
creative praxes that generate and modify habits. However, Bourdieu and colleagues pay little empirical attention to children or the precise processes of that
early cultural practice, instead largely outsourcing those explanations back to
socialization and the internalization concept (Garnier 2015), as well as pointing
to formal education as a strategy through which families can reproduce their
social position in subsequent generations (Thomson 2008). Despite documenting in detail the processes of remodeling a secondary habitus through a boxing
gym (Wacquant 2004), for example, Wacquant (2016) describes the process of
acquiring the primary habitus vaguely as occurring "through osmosis" in the
family microcosm (68). Thus Bourdieu and his contemporaries leave open a theoretical space for childhood theorists to grapple with.

Indeed, because of childhood's relevance to Bourdieu's theory of habitus, a
number of child development and education scholars have elaborated Bour-
dieuian theory to understand aspects of childhood and schooling within
broader cultural and structural contexts (Miller and Goodnow 1995; Alanen,
Brooker, and Mayall 2015; Connolly 2004). A large emphasis has been on recon-
stituting Bourdieu's (1977) concern with patriarchal relations of power within
intergenerational analyses of social change and dominance hegemonies that
structure and maintain inequalities between adults and children (Miller and
Goodnow 1995). For example, Vuorisalo and Alanen (2015) analyze how preschool
children use strategies to acquire and deploy different forms of capital in negotiation with teachers, and how this unequal distribution of capital results in an

unrecognized, stratified social order—a form of symbolic violence. A second prominent theme has been the effects produced by incongruities between the forms of habitus generated in different fields, whether it is the impact of differences between home and school habitus on educational achievement (Connolly 2004) or parent-child negotiations (Mayall 2015), or how conflicts between local and globalizing ideas about childhood shape children's dispositions for work and labor practices (André and Hilgers 2015).

I extend these ideas in this book, considering how new kinds of health services, ideologies, changing demographics, and patterns of morbidity and mortality can contribute to new kinds of struggles in the field and through new practices restructure forms of habitus for the children who negotiate these changes in school contexts. The emphasis in childhood scholarship, though, tends to be on how children negotiate interpersonal relations, or how changing social and political-economic environments engender generational differences in dispositions. Less attention is paid to the processes through which children collectively produce cultural meanings and practices, how they use those meanings and practices to navigate intergenerational, institutional, and political-economic constraints, and how the embodiment of such practices helps to reproduce inequalities. In this book, I use a view of children's socially structured cultural production to reveal, for example, how children establish and embody practices of "not hungry" rather than accept stigmatized provisions, or how children construct an understanding of rheumatic fever etiology that shapes their perceptions of risk and subsequent practices of accessing health care. This understanding of children's collective cultural production comes out of a different way of conceptualizing childhood learning: the shift in thinking brought by the developmental psychologists who laid the groundwork for Corsaro's (1992) model of interpretive reproduction.

Developmental Psychology and Interpretive Reproduction

The constructivist approach of developmental psychology challenged the determinism of early socialization theory, instead emphasizing the child's active role in socialization processes. If, as Corsaro (2015) puts it, for the social determinists, society appropriates the child, then for the constructivist developmental psychologists, it is the child who appropriates society, albeit still primarily through processes of internalization.

Of great significance from this era is the work of psychologists Jean Piaget (1967) and Lev Vygotsky (1978), the latter of whom directly influenced Corsaro's (1992) model of interpretive reproduction. Piaget has been the more well known, although he began writing in the 1920s and it took several decades for his work to gain influence. By the 1960s, Piaget's theories dominated developmental psychology. His legacy is the view of children as active participants in their development and the argument that, from infancy, children interpret, organize, and use information from their environment to construct conceptions (mental structures or schema) of their physical and social worlds (Ginsburg and Opper 1988). This is a process that primarily occurs inside individual children's heads, constrained by the biological development of cognitive structures. Cognitive development in Piaget's view therefore occurs from the "inside out" (Burman, as cited in Connolly 2004), first in the individual minds and then expressed "outside" through activity and behavior.

By contrast, Vygotsky (1978) situates children's development within their collective actions and interactions set within society. Development, in this view, instead occurs from the "outside in," whereby a child first experiences the world as an actor embedded within culture and social relations, and these interactions then become internalized as mental schemes of social and physical systems (Connolly 2004). Language is therefore a critical part of children's development, first used to communicate with others, and then as internal speech or thought used for self-regulation and consciousness (Smith 2013). The significance of this process for learning is captured in the "zone of proximal development" concept, whereby through social interaction children can engage in more complex forms of activity and behavior than what they could understand or accomplish on their own (Vygotsky 1978). While Piaget saw children's capacities as limited by the biological architecture of brain development, for Vygotsky the limitations can be found in what, when, and with whom children experience, or what more recent scholars have termed the quality and quantity of "scaffolding" others make available to the child to support them in stretching their capacities (Smith 2013).

Although Vygotsky died in 1934, his work became influential in Western scholarship only from the 1960s and 1970s, and in recent decades has been particularly taken up in education fields. For example, Paul Connolly (2004), who tackles the increasingly global question of boys' underachievement at school, finds value in Vygotsky's attention to the social nature of learning, which has particular relevance for children's developing ideas of gender and class. However, Connolly develops Vygotsky's work further by considering how children's socially learned ideas and behavior are influenced and shaped by cultural contexts and differential relations of power embedded in much broader communities, incorporating insights from Bourdieu and Elias. While scholars in the Vygotskyan tradition typically focus on simplified two-way interactions between a child and one other individual, using Elias's (1978) "figuration" concept Connolly locates children within open, interdependent networks of relations that, crucially, are infused with differential relations of power that create systems of dominance and determine which ideas are established as norms. Connolly then finds common ground between Vygotsky and Bourdieu in the processes of internalization; the way that cognitive schemes, once internalized, form the habitus that structures future action and reflects the particular contexts and broader social structures of children's lived experience.

The work of both Vygotsky and Connolly, however, still remains uncritical of the reliance on internalization as the key mechanism of cultural production and learning, which limits children's activities to the acquisition of adult culture and practices, measuring child competencies and understandings against an adult standard and emphasizing outcomes over processes. Corsaro (1992), while heavily influenced by Vygotsky's notions of children's development as collective and interactional, constructed his model of interpretive reproduction by extending processes of social reproduction beyond simply internalization to include children's appropriation, innovation, and creative interpretation of culture. Like Vygotsky, Corsaro breaks away from theories of socialization that position the child as individually and privately internalizing the skills, knowledge, and culture of adults in a linear fashion. Instead, Corsaro views childhood socialization as a collective, social process where children remake culture anew.

Using the metaphor of an orb spider web, Corsaro (2015) describes how children work from the family unit, represented at the center of the web, and collectively spin spirals of peer cultures across the spokes of the web, which represent different fields or locales that compose various social institutions (such as family, educational, and religious institutions). Through these peer cultures, knowledge and practices are produced and reproduced, and gradually develop into forms that enable participation in the adult world. Focusing on play within children's peer groups, Corsaro describes how children appropriate adult cultural frameworks and routines and transform these into variations, for example through "keying," in which a new activity is modeled on the patterning of an existing activity, or through "embellishments," in which certain elements of routines are intensified through repetition or exaggeration.

Interpretive reproduction offers a way of viewing children as significant contributors to health through their collective production of cultural meanings and practices—for example, the way that children construct novel concepts of sore throat, or the ways that adult frames of death influence but are not duplicated in the way children themselves employ death concepts and language. While Corsaro's model is strong on agency, it is, as James (2013) notes, weak on constraint. *Structure* is present, represented in the spokes of the orb web around which children spin spirals of meaning. But children's activities are not a free-for-all of endless possibility, and the model does not capture the particularities of how these structures guide children's cultural production: how options are constrained by relations of authority or resource availability; how the body itself structures cultural production as the material substrate through which sociality is enacted and embodied; and, to paraphrase Clifford Geertz (1973), how children become caught in the webs of meaning they themselves have spun.

In this book I therefore aim to work in the gap between Corsaro and Bourdieu, detailing the way children's interpretive practices articulate with both the biological structures of a body and the constraints of material deprivation and institutional and societal structures. I argue that these processes are best captured by a coproduction framework that makes room for children's agency by positioning them in dialectical relationship with the body and society, each reinforcing, remodeling, or transforming the other. Conceptualizing children's activities as a coproduction shifts the view of interpretive reproduction from webs made from children's spirals creatively freewheeling over adult spokes, to one where children's cultural meanings and practices are constrained and enabled by experiences of the body and wider social systems, while those meanings and practices simultaneously mediate how those wider social systems work on bodies. Coproduction also means that children, in negotiating the structures of their childhoods, collectively create new cultural forms within peer groups that not only help to structure their own habitus, but also leave open the possibility for children to modify the habitus of their parents as well.

Why Is the Body Important?

In many studies of biological or medical anthropology, children's bodies have represented important physical records of environments and events experienced, encoded in measurable processes of growth, development and repair, biochemistry and disease (Flinn 1999; Horton and Barker 2010; Littleton 2007; Panter-Brick 1998a; Panter-Brick, Todd, and Baker 1996). The role of the body in these studies is to provide a map for the distribution and dynamics of power and resources within and across populations (Krieger 2005). However, the body is not only the material substrate upon which structural inequities leave their marks, but the locus of experience (Merleau-Ponty 1962) and of practice (Bourdieu 1984)—the sites at which the structured world is converted into social meanings and translated into practices. Children's interpretations are important mediators of their own health because their practices have real physical effects. For humans, the embodiment of inequity, therefore, involves not only the biological processes of converting energy to growth, immune function, and homeostasis, but also experiences of the body incarnate (Frankenberg 1990) made meaningful in different ways within unequal social worlds.

The body already underpins childhood, which is socially constructed around a universal period of biological immaturity, the significance of which is culturally variable (James and Prout 1990; Prout 2000b). In the West, this immaturity is conflated with social vulnerability and incompetence, producing childhoods characterized by a prolonged period of dependence and restriction. In other places, such as southeastern Mexico (Kramer 2005), and Java and Nepal (Nag,

White, Peet, et al. 1978), incomplete growth does not preclude the expectation of being a full and contributing member of society, and children's labor activities can form an essential part of domestic and community economic life. Within this period of growth also sit a number of reasonably canalized biological life events to which variable degrees of significance may be socially ascribed by adults and children. The eruption and loss of teeth are socially celebrated by the tooth fairy in North America (Clark 1998) or mark a new life stage for the Ngoni children of Malawi (Read 1968). Whereas Davis and Davis (1989) suggest there was virtually no adolescence in traditional rural Morocco as onset of puberty was quickly followed by marriage and the conferring of adulthood, in Aotearoa and elsewhere in the West, neurological science is used to extend the stage of perceived immaturity up to 25, with a host of subsequent policies and interventions (France 2012).

The body, therefore, bears important social markers that differentiate and transform social experiences across societies, just as these experiences in turn transform bodies. These markers of growth, however, along with other universal but culturally variegated bodily experiences—illness, injury, fatigue, emotion, stress, hunger—are *biosocially* produced; the underlying biology itself is underwritten by cultural processes that mediate how these experiences are distributed and interpreted. Thus, sociologist Chris Shilling (1993) describes the relationship between the body and culture as *dialectical*—a coproduction in which each simultaneously helps to produce the other.

Shilling's ideas developed from Turner's (1984, 1992) concern that sociological treatments of the body have tended to fall into either biological or cultural reductionism, what he terms "foundationalist" and "anti-foundationalist" approaches. Foundationalist approaches assume the body as a material object, distinct from the social, while anti-foundationalist approaches claim that it is not possible to make a distinction between the body and its representations, since we have access to the materiality of the body only through the discourses that structure and shape it. Turner proposes a reconciliation of these two approaches by way of "methodological eclecticism" (Prout 2000a, 4): acknowledging the value and intellectual validity of both approaches, and seeing them as complementary. Shilling (1993), however, argues that combining the two approaches "without altering any of their basic parameters" (103) is not theoretically coherent and that it is the relationships between the body and society that are critical. He therefore proposes a framework that takes the body as a social and biological work in progress throughout the life course, with each resourcing and constraining the other: a dialectic coproduction. For example, Shilling describes the embodiment of social gender inequalities that occurs when average biological sex differences are socially highlighted and transformed into absolute and naturalized gender differences.[10] The subsequent socialization toward particular patterns of behavior further reinforces those differences—for example, encouraging men to build muscle mass and women to maintain small bodies. The biological and the cultural thus work together to mutually coproduce both the body and society.

Despite the importance of childhood as the foundational stage of this biosocial development, Shilling's (1993) discussion of childhood is limited to chapters on Elias and Bourdieu, in which children are positioned as passive receptacles of socialization and "civilizing." Instead, sociologist Alan Prout (2000b, 2005) builds on Shilling's thinking to theorize the dynamic relationship between the body and culture in childhood and to challenge the biosocial dualism that had separated the social constructivists from the developmental scientists. In this view, the body is the site of children's experience, and their environments both structure and are structured around their bodies; children are therefore hybrids of their biological inheritance and the social world, which together mediate children's cultural and biological development. This is an understanding that has long been present in anthropology: Boas's early recognition of the biocultural nature of developmental plasticity set the stage for a proliferation of cultural studies of childhood (Boas 1974 [1911]; cf. Montgomery 2009), in which the molding and disciplining of children's bodies in culturally patterned ways is a main feature of socialization (e.g., Geurts 2003), while child-rearing practices are configured around the biology of infant bodies (LeVine 1977). This attention to the body carried through to the interpretive childhood anthropology of the early 1990s, which further located the body within children's experiences and understandings of identity and illness (e.g., Christensen 1999; James 1993). However, Prout's notion that children (and therefore adults) develop within a dialectical "medley of culture and nature" opens up a space to conceptualize the role children play in the production of their own bodies—bodies not only as made by adults and experienced by children, but also as a coproduction between children and society, biology and culture, agency and constraint.

Prout's work has sparked new theoretical interest in the hybridity concept: to break down nature/culture binaries in childhood studies (Kraftl 2013; Ryan 2012), navigate the biopolitics of childhood (Lee and Motzkau 2011), reassert children as biological creatures within a changing environment that has particular effects upon those biologies (Lee 2013), and open up childhood studies to more cross-pollination with the psycho-biological disciplines (Thorne 2007). Very little of this recent work has been ethnographic, although Davies (2015) emphasizes the embodied sensory and interphysical nature of children's family relationships in a context of socioeconomic deprivation in central England, showing for example, how children monitor the bodies of younger siblings for care needs and negotiate power hierarchies through physical confrontation. Still missing, however, are ethnographic accounts of how children coproduce their bodies in relationship with society, and how these biosocial processes of the body and its interpretation unfold, temporally and in context.

What then, are these processes through which children co-construct, reproduce, internalize, and embody their worlds? How are children's health practices
structured by institutions, state interventions, wider cultural discourses, and
material resources? How does material deprivation become translated into interpretive practices of the body—a habitus of childhood inequality? How do children
negotiate, accommodate, and embody structural vulnerability produced by
their social positioning? And how does the instability and risk wrought by
structural violence become woven into children's cultural production?

These are the questions I will address through the remainder of this book.
They are questions less about what children experience and more about what
children *do*—though, of course, children's practices derive from their experiences.
Importantly, these questions point to why what children do *matters*—suggesting
that the child who is invisible in policy is very much active in the coproduction of
their health. These perspectives reveal children who are actively negotiating
unstable, constrained worlds, but worlds that are in part produced by children
themselves, as they collectively translate their material conditions and cohabi-
tants into cultural meanings, social relationships, and embodied practices, at the
same time as they are shaped and constrained by those conditions. As economic
inequalities stamp biology with signatures of poverty—respiratory illness, dental
decay, stress—the state targets these young bodies; and through their experiences
of health interventions in the institution, children construct new understandings
of illness and generate new practices of the body. This is a view of how children
co-create their habitus, working creatively within structures that open up or constrain opportunities and resources, and in doing so help to generate the habitus
that in turn guides future practice.

Overview of Chapters

I address these questions through the following chapters. In chapter 2, I establish
the world of Tūrama School, both through broader political-economic, historical, and societal perspectives and also as seen through children's own eyes.
This institutional environment, shaped by local, national, and global forces,
sets the structures that children negotiate and transform in the coproduction of
their health.

Chapter 3 sets out the main power structure operating within the school:
the separation of adult staff and child pupils, which explicitly works on children's
bodies differently from adults. I keenly felt the dynamics at work here as a
researcher whose adult body transgressed these boundaries and inadvertently
revealed the power of these forces. In this chapter I discuss how such institutional structures challenge the role of the researcher who attempts to balance
what are sometimes competing ethical obligations to children and adults, and I

propose the role of "transparent guest" as a guide for navigating between adult and child worlds and their associated rules and expectations.

Having established the geographic, social, historical, and political economic contexts for this book and the methodological complexities within which the data were produced, over the following five chapters I unpack the dynamics of health coproduction for children at Tūrama School to answer the question, How do children participate in the coproduction of their health? I take the case of the school rheumatic fever prevention clinic and related campaign as my point of entry in chapter 4, showing how children collectively create cultural meanings of illness and health-care routines around the clinic in ways unanticipated by policy makers. Children's embodied interpretations of illness and creative practices mediate their engagement with health care and pharmaceuticals and are key ways that children shape their health in coproduction with health-care services.

In chapter 5 I consider how children coproduce their health together with state discourses of responsibility. Focusing on public debates around the provisioning of school lunches, I describe how children contribute to their dietary patterns by making social meanings and practices around different kinds of food, shaped by wider discourses and material constraint. In chapter 6, this material deprivation becomes translated into interpretive practices of the body to form a habitus of childhood inequality that in turn orients future practice. I argue that structural constraints on resources or power shape the degree to which children tune in to particular bodily signals that tell children they are cold, hungry, or sick. At the same time, children's peer cultures produce socially accepted meanings and practices that further reinforce how those signals are experienced in the body.

In chapter 7 I explore how the instability wrought by economic and housing policy is translated into children's practices of resilience, and how the interconnected and embodied nature of these practices contributes to children's health. I draw on socio-ecological frameworks for resilience that reconcile children's structural vulnerability with their competence as social actors by placing the child within broader social and physical environments that constrain their activities or provide resources for children to use. Finally, in chapter 8 I consider how children coproduce their health in relation to the structural violence that mediates their experiences of death. Tūrama School children's "small talk of death" can reveal their experiences of a social positioning where they are thrice marginalized by their ethnic, socioeconomic, and age statuses, the confluence of which creates a context where death is both common and culturally salient. While children collectively compile understandings of what death means and the likelihood that it will affect them, adults invoking death, for example in health promotion, inadvertently tap into a powerful expressive device of children, both reinforcing a sense of fear and urgency around death and also shaping children's practices of health care.

Together, these chapters illustrate how the coproduction of children's health occurs within peer ecologies, grounded in the body and guided by wider institutional and societal structures that children translate into their own collective meanings and practices. I conclude in chapter 9 by reflecting on the implications for theory and practice of conceptualizing child health in this way: beginning with the *children* in child health and taking seriously their role in a coproduction between interconnected, embodied individuals, making meanings from their experiences of a structured world, collectively practicing childhood.

2

The World of Tūrama School

In one of my first conversations with Ruby, she asks me if I want to be in a gang.

"Uh, no," I say, emphatically.

"I want to be in a gang when I grow up," Ruby tells me. Her father is in a gang. "I want to be like my dad. I don't want to be like my mum, she does nuffink all day."

"Is there anyone else you could be like?" I ask hopefully, and Ruby pauses, thinking.

"Mm, there's my auntie. She works at Countdown,"[1] she says dubiously. "But I think being in a gang would be better."

While teachers described Ruby's gang-member father as a scary man, I could see why they tended to have a soft spot for Ruby. Mrs. Randall, who taught her in year five (age nine), told me she initially thought Ruby was slow, she was so withdrawn. By year six, the green-eyed, ruddy-cheeked Ruby had elbowed her way into position as the undisputed leader of the girls in her class. "She's the boss of us. She's like our mum," her friend Marielle tells me one day, explaining how she and the other girls have to ask Ruby if they want to go to the toilet, because she wants to know where they are going "or else we might get hurt." As a ten-year-old, Ruby is bold, insightful, and, although I once spotted her changing her times-tables score from a 98 to a 100, academically confident.

I don't believe Ruby at first when she tells me she lives with eighteen other people, because she can play with the truth at times; she made up a "fake" birthday in December because, she later rationalized, she shares her June birthday with an uncle and wanted her own day. But she draws me a map of the six bedrooms where her grandparents, parents, siblings, aunts, and cousins live, plus the sitting room where two uncles sleep. Another auntie stayed the other night, too, because the police were down the road looking for synthetics (drugs), and her auntie was scared—she had been to jail before. To be sure, I later checked the story with her teacher, Mrs. Charles, who said, "That sounds about right." Mrs. Charles knows a lot about her pupil's home lives, and she has given Ruby her phone number in case she needs it one day.

Ruby's circumstances, while not those of an average Tūrama School child, are unusual more for the size of the rental home rather than the people-to-bedroom ratio. Her friend Mila similarly shares a bedroom with three brothers. Ruby's childhood is, however, far from the average New Zealand childhood. Data from the 2013 census show the average household size is 3.5 people in Ruby's suburb, well above the national average of 2.7 (Statistics New Zealand 2015). The crowded conditions likely have various impacts on the family's health, not least of which is stress; Ruby describes living with so many people as "full" and "annoying, 'cause there's a lot of arguing." In an English context, Hayley Davies (2015) found that her child participants experienced overcrowded homes as stressful. Also in this house, Ruby's young cousin developed rheumatic fever, which is linked to overcrowding (Jaine, Baker, and Venugopal 2011), and he now receives the same monthly prophylactic penicillin injections as Victor, whom we met in chapter 1.

Tūrama School represents children at the most deprived end of the socioeconomic scale, childhoods geographically bounded to the extent that, until recent media attention, the deep inequalities differentiating New Zealand childhoods were nearly invisible to the middle class. These deprived childhoods also disproportionately belong to Māori and Pasifika children (Henare, Puckey, and Nicholson 2011; Perry 2016). Aotearoa is a multi-ethnic nation located in the Pacific and administered by dominant British colonial systems of governance in partnership with the indigenous Māori peoples. Since World War II, high numbers of Polynesian migrants have come to settle particularly in the South Auckland region alongside urban Māori, and Auckland is now often referred to as the Polynesian capital of the world (Barbera 2011). In Aotearoa, these Māori and Pasifika childhoods are configured around Western legal, political-economic, institutional, and social frameworks of childhood that see non-Pākehā[2] children as deviations from the norm, historically represented as novelties for tourists or as mortality statistics, as problems to be "Europeanized" or children who need "catching up" to Pākehā level (May 2001). Māori childhoods are colonized childhoods, and a misalignment between indigenous and Pākehā conceptions of childhood and practices of child-rearing, embedded in law, policy, and institutions and compounded by neoliberal economic and housing policies, has perpetuated inequities and cultural alienation for children like those at Tūrama School. These are the other, the *othered* Aotearoa childhoods: bicultural childhoods, childhoods in poverty.

From the perspective of Tūrama School children living them, however, these are normal childhoods filled with fun, freedom, and lots of love, even if sometimes things are not so great, like when Ruby worries that her dad will get shot, or when Whetu gets taken away from his mum, or when Arya gets teased for being poor, even though she is definitely not. The census data that demonstrate the ethnic composition and relative poverty of Tūrama School children constitute only one representation of a lifeworld that is understood quite differently by those living within it.

Yet economic insecurity, neoliberal reform, cultural dissonance, and the legacies of colonization and migration histories have all contributed to the conditions of Tūrama School childhoods, even if these factors remain outside the children's field of view. Historical and contemporary housing, economic, health, and social policies shape both the marginalized circumstances of the children's families and also the institution's role in mediating the harmful impacts. The discourses, practices, and interventions of families and the institution in response to economic insecurity comprise the structures that Tūrama School children negotiate, reconstruct, and transform in the coproduction of their health.

In this chapter, I aim to set the scene for the analysis of children's health understandings and practices to follow by outlining the major structural features of Tūrama School childhoods that form the context for their health coproduction. As the central question of this book requires a view of how children come to understand health through their own embodied perspectives, I represent Tūrama School childhoods as they are viewed from historical, political, and societal perspectives—the researcher's view—but also as they are viewed by Tūrama School children themselves. I consider the geographic and ethnic composition of Papakura, where Tūrama School is located, and how this translates into children's perceptions of their world, as well as the impacts of economic inequities that leave 290,000 Aotearoa children in poverty. These inequities are shaped by colonization and migration histories, and so have significant implications for Māori and Pasifika health; rheumatic fever in particular represents an important contemporary manifestation of eroding housing and economic conditions in South Auckland that can be traced to historical circumstances. Finally, I outline the historical and present roles of the New Zealand state and school institutions in caring for children's health and welfare—roles that directly shape Tūrama School children's health experiences in the classroom.

What Culture Are You?

The children of Tūrama School have been relegated to an area of highest deprivation within Papakura, South Auckland, through the doubly marginalizing intersection of social class and ethnicity—the result of historical colonization and migration events compounded by contemporary neoliberal policy. Formerly recognized as its own city and later as its own district, since the amalgamation of cities into the Auckland super city, Papakura is now officially designated as a local board area, with a population of around 45,000. Locals call themselves a town. In this town there is literally a wrong side of the tracks, a train line dividing low-quality state housing from new developments that attract middle-class commuters as a housing crisis drives up prices in the central city. This class segregation is also highly correlated with ethnicity. Māori represented 28 percent of the Papakura population in the 2013 census—making for the third highest Māori population in Auckland—and Pacific peoples represented about 14.5 percent of the Papakura population. However, local school rolls show a further clustering of ethnic populations; more than 70 percent of children at Tūrama School are Māori (although many of this group have Pasifika and/or European heritage), and around 20 percent are of Pacific Island descent.[3] Although Pākehā, or New Zealand European people, are the majority ethnic group in Papakura as well as nationally, fewer than 4 percent of Tūrama School children identify as Pākehā. Meanwhile, schools in more affluent areas of Papakura tend to have few children of Māori or Pacific descent—less than 10 percent—and higher numbers of Asian and Indian immigrants as well as a Pākehā majority.

Growing up as they are in an ethnic enclave, then, most Tūrama School children's experiences are of being a majority ethnic group. I quickly became aware of this when I was repeatedly asked, "What culture are you?" by children who had difficulty placing me within their emic ethnic classification system. I could not give any answer that satisfied them—something I had never experienced as a privileged member of the country's majority Pākehā ethnic group. While "Māori" and "Pākehā" are terms constituted in relation to each other— the hapū (subtribes) and iwi (tribes) of Aotearoa, and the European explorers and settlers who arrived following James Cook's voyage (Bell 2004)—these children did not hold a concept of my identity as Pākehā, let alone much sense of the colonial implications of my Pākehā status in relation to themselves. If I told them I was Pākehā, they were embarrassed; many of them used "Pākehā" to refer to light-skinned Māori, but the term carried a derogatory valence. If I said I was a New Zealander, they were confused. Some children thought that I was Māori, and one girl asked me if I was Samoan. Others decided that I was Scottish, English, or Irish. I came to realize that "culture," as these children are using it, indexes ancestry via country of origin, but constructed in such a way as to avoid the racial politics salient in their peer groups.

I register the concern with country of origin while observing the school clinic one day, when a boy who is waiting for his turn to see the nurse asks me, "What culture are you?"

"Pākehā," I say.

"No, you're not."

"Yeah, I am," I say, not all that surprised by this stage.

"No, you're Irish."

"I'm not Irish."

"You're lying."

"I'm not lying."

"You are lying. You're Irish. You have white skin. People with white skin are from . . . where are white people from?"

Based on the vague notion that lightly pigmented people originate from Ireland (or Scotland), children therefore explained my "culture" as Irish or Scottish. While Pākehā New Zealanders typically conflate cultural and ethnic identity with nationality and emphasize country of birth—identifying as New Zealander rather than British—Tūrama School children's cultural classification system emphasizes different core properties: ancestry, perhaps influenced by the salience of *whakapapa* (genealogy) in *Te Ao Māori* (the Māori world). They then apply the same logic to white people that white people would apply to everyone else—the children of Pacific or Asian ancestry identify and are identified as Tongan, Samoan, or Chinese, even when they or their parents were born in New Zealand; by that logic, white people should be identified by their ancestral origins, rather than their place of birth. Hence I, having mostly English ancestry, should identify as English.

I had an opportunity to expand my emerging sense of how Tūrama School children saw the world when I spent the day in Mrs. Stevens' class. Charismatic, opinionated, and with a uniquely laid-back teaching style, Mrs. Stevens has a disdain for "political correctness"; she does not hesitate to call children "retards" or "juvenile delinquents," and she describes her class as "special" (insinuating "special needs"). Yet boys who rebel against their own teachers and are frequently disciplined for behavioral problems will come up to talk with Mrs. Stevens. This year, all of the children who had truancy issues were placed into Mrs. Stevens' class so that they could be managed together, and so far all of those children have been coming to school. Mrs. Stevens jokes that she wouldn't mind if some of them were truant more often, encouraging one exasperating boy to take a day off to give her a break.

For me, Mrs. Stevens' class often provided a window into the worlds of these children through her practice of promoting free and open conversation. She begins each day by discussing items in the news, which can prompt very long digressions; discussion of a news item about twins who were separated at birth ended up with a long laugh over photos of dogs that look like their owners. As part of these open discussions, children will make comments that reflect their worlds without the censorship that is usually maintained in the presence of adults. Children will share their knowledge of drugs: "I saw Mr. McPherson's son smoking a lazy tinny" (marijuana joint); childbirth: "when you shit the baby out"; and gang affiliations: "Mozart is in a wolf gang, aye, Miss? Yeah, like the Killer Beez."

Mrs. Stevens was also very happy to hold class discussions about issues relevant to my work. When I expressed an interest in finding out more about the children's perceptions of the ethnic breakdown of the country, we spontaneously decide to co-investigate this, integrating the teaching of percentages as the math learning for the day. With the children lounging on the mat in front of the whiteboard, Mrs. Stevens takes them through a basic tutorial about percentages. Then I draw a long vertical rectangle on the board, divided into tenths and labeled from 0 percent to 100 percent.

"So, if this box is all of the kids at our school, where would I color up to, to show all of the children under fifteen years old?" I ask.

"You'd color to the 100," the children correctly reply.

"And if I wanted to show how many children are under four years old?"

"Zero," they reply.

"What about if I wanted to show how many are girls?"

"About to the 50," they say.

"Let's do something a bit harder," I say, and Mrs. Stevens steps in.

"How about how many children are Māori?" she asks. This question elicits a range of answers, including eleven-year-old Navahn's facetious assertion that most children were Pākehā. "What are you talking about, Navahn?" Mrs. Stevens waves her arms. "Do you see mostly Pākehā in here? There's Chloe. That's it."

"Who here is Māori?" she continues. "Put your hand down, Joy, you're Islander. Jasper, Trystan, put your hands up, you're Māori. Paula . . ." Mrs. Stevens squints at the small girl in front of her. "I'm pretty sure you're Māori."

"I'm Samoan," says Paula.

"You can be both," I say. I am not sure why either of us are defining the children's ethnicity for them.

"So apart from an identity crisis, what we've worked out here is that about 70 percent of you are Māori," Mrs. Stevens announces. She turns to me. "Which is about the school's average?"

"Yeah, or just over, I think." I draw the line on the board in between the 70 and 75 and shade in the box, then add the shading for Pacific Islander (20 percent) and "other" (Asian and Pākehā: 5 percent).

"OK, so here's a question," I say. "What if we make this box every person in New Zealand. How many are girls?" The class decides just over 50 percent—they have heard that women live longer than men. "OK, so how much do you think we would color in to show the number of people who are Māori?"

"Ninety percent!" A child shouts. "Seventy percent! Eighty! About fifty?"

"Remembering that this school is 72 percent Māori," I say to the children who were calling out high numbers. "Ninety-five percent," they shout. I put marks along the box showing all the guesses. Most of them are above 75 percent. Navahn's guess of 45 percent is by far the lowest.

"Are you ready to find out who was closest?" I ask. "I'm going to show you the answer." I hold my pen near the top of the box, and with dramatic effect gradually drop the pen lower and lower along the scale while the children gasp, to stop at around 15 percent. "This is how many people in New Zealand are Māori," I say. The children gape at me. I color in the box to show Pākehā and other ethnic groups.

Seeing their astonishment, Mrs. Stevens explains. "See, the thing is, you guys live very insulated lives. Most of you have never even been out of Papakura! You look around you and think this is what everywhere looks like." She tells us the story of when she arrived in Papakura and wondered where all the white people were. "You think me and Julie and Chloe are the minorities, but actually we're the majority in New Zealand!"

"You guys are actually really rare," I say. "You're special."

"Well, we already knew this class was special," Mrs. Stevens jokes.

"It's funny," I comment to Mrs. Stevens, "I suspected this was what they thought, but I also thought maybe—because they watch a lot of TV—that they would've picked up that Papakura looked different."

"But TV isn't reality," she points out. "This . . ." she gestures around the class. "Is reality."

"Shall we do one more question?" I ask her. "Can we do a bit of a controversial one?"

"You know me!" Mrs. Stevens replies. "Of course we can do a controversial one." I have done this exercise a couple of times in interviews with children, so I have an inkling of what to expect. I draw a horizontal line on the board and mark it from one to ten. "On this line, ten is the richest people in New Zealand, and one is the poorest."

"Oooh," says Mrs. Stevens.

"Thinking about the kids who go to our school, on average, where do you think this school is?"

"Nine!" One child shouts. A range of numbers come in, most between four and nine. One girl chooses two, and Mrs. Stevens nods at her. "You're quite onto it today, aren't you, Joy?"

I have started to feel uncomfortable. "I haven't quite thought this through," I mumble to Mrs. Stevens. "Now we have to give them the answer."

"That's OK," she brushes off my concern. "What is the answer?"

"I was thinking school deciles," I said. "As a good proxy for the community."

"Oh, yup," she says, and proceeds to explain the school decile rating system. "So every school is given a number based on things like how many people in the community are on benefits, how many people don't have a job, how many people need state housing." I notice she is naming concrete things that would be familiar to these children. "If you don't have many of these things in your community, then you're a ten, and if you have lots, you're a one. So, what do you guys think we are?" The children's responses don't really change from what was given previously.

Mrs. Stevens circles the one, and the class falls quiet. "You guys are ones," she says. The children are wide-eyed, blinking.

"Well," I hasten to add, "Schools that are ones still have some families who are rich, and schools that are tens have some families that are poor. And you guys actually have a really good school. What schools do you think get the most money from the government?"

"The tens?" Someone guesses.

"No, the ones. I went to a ten school, and we didn't have tablets."

"Yeah," Mrs. Stevens adds, "we had to buy our own tablets for my kids. And you know what, you guys are ones now, but aim for a ten! Your parents are ones but you don't have to be. Work hard, get your education, and go be tens!"

Despite this speech, the children are subdued, staring, processing. "They're so quiet," I comment to Mrs. Stevens, and she laughs. "Yeah, look, you're all depressed now that we've burst your little bubbles."

I wipe the graphs off the board and a child asks, "Can you ask us more questions?"

"Yeah," Mrs. Stevens says with a wink at me. "Next time Julie's in our class we'll ask more questions."

While this school and community are far from what might be considered "mainstream" New Zealand and represent the extreme end of the socioeconomic scale in census data, what I took from this day was how normal this community and this school are from the perspectives of the children living there. This normalcy is despite the visibility of media discourses about child poverty and media representations of New Zealand lifestyles that are very different from the children's own. This is the world for Tūrama School children, and this is the normal world.

Unequal Childhoods

The struggles of Tūrama School families have until recently been largely rendered invisible by the dominant cultural zeitgeist, which reflects a nostalgic imagining of Aotearoa childhoods as happy, protected, resource-rich, and world-leading (Tap 2007). According to the Child Poverty Monitor, 27 percent (approximately 290,000) of New Zealand children are now considered to live in poverty, meaning they live in households with incomes less than 60 percent of the contemporary median after housing costs (Duncanson, Oben, McGee, et al. 2017). International pressure has provoked serious attention to the issue of childhood deprivation. As a signatory to the United Nations 2030 Agenda for sustainable development, which came into effect in January 2016, New Zealand is required to halve, from a 2015 baseline, the rates of children from zero to seventeen years old living in poverty (United Nations 2015). Childhood inequity in Aotearoa has also been an increasing concern of researchers who document the short- and long-term effects of poverty on health, education, and crime (Baker, Barnard, Kvalsvig, et al. 2012; Boston and Chapple 2014; Fergusson, Horwood, and Boden 2008; Gibb, Fergusson, and Horwood 2012; Pearce and Dorling 2006; Rashbrooke 2013). This body of research includes three ongoing major longitudinal studies of child health: the Dunedin Multidisciplinary Health and Development Study, now on the second generation (Poulton, Moffitt, and Silva 2015; Silva 1990); the Christchurch Health and Development study of children born in 1977 (Fergusson, Boden, and Horwood 2015); and the Growing Up in New Zealand study, which began in 2010 (Morton, Atatoa Carr, Grant, et al. 2013), all of which demonstrate links between early childhood environments and life trajectory. Another major longitudinal study of Pacific families in Aotearoa, initiated in 2000, investigates links between a host of developmental pathways and health outcomes for Pasifika children, including culturally nuanced perspectives on the impacts of gambling, nutrition, alcohol consumption, and violence on child health (Savila, Sundborn, Hirao, et al. 2011).

As child and adult morbidity and mortality statistics testify against the beloved cultural myth of an egalitarian society, action groups and the media have also drawn increasing attention to the numbers of children living below the poverty line, investigating, for example, inequalities in child educational achievement (Johnston 2015), housing conditions (Johnston and Knox 2017), and what children have for lunch (Barraclough 2017). Child poverty became a further issue in the 2017 election, and under pressure from the left-leaning opposition, during a debate the incumbent National Party leader made a surprise pledge to lift 100,000 children out of poverty within the next six years (Radio New Zealand 2017). This represented a major concession by a party that, up until that point, had disagreed with opposition parties, the Children's Commissioner, researchers, experts, and diverse organizations and action groups about the extent of and ability to measure child poverty in New Zealand (Peters and Besley 2014; Rashbrooke 2017). The struggles of impoverished adults, however, were rarely mentioned. In a neoliberal society where poverty is routinely discounted with discourses of individual responsibility (Boston and Chapple 2014), children, as the innocent and vulnerable faces of the future, represent the one group who cannot be held responsible for their circumstances and thus headline appeals for policy change.

The children of Tūrama School are not immune from these discourses; they see the news, and so they, too, are concerned for these children living in poverty, perhaps in Africa, or with those homeless people they see on the street. Ten-year-old Amberlee does not like Prime Minister John Key, she tells me, because he puts up the prices of the houses so the poor people can't buy them. You can tell if someone is poor, she explains, because they don't shave their face and cart their things around in a trolley on the street, and poor children don't have beds so they have to sleep on the floor in leaky houses. On a one-to-ten scale of poorest to richest, Amberlee guesses the children at Tūrama School are about a four, which means that on Monday and Tuesday you might bring lunch, but on Wednesday and Friday you have none. And some children, like this one girl, Helen, have no proper shoes and holes in their clothes.

Amberlee is particularly observant, and her guess is one of the more accurate that children shared with me; whether I asked individuals, small groups, or entire classes like Mrs. Stevens', few rated Tūrama School less than five, and many thought they were a nine or a ten. Tūrama School straddles two suburbs that, according to the New Zealand Index of Multiple Deprivation, are in the 97th percentile for deprivation nationally, characterized by families with low median income, low frequency of educational qualifications, and high levels of government assistance benefits. Often, two or three families occupy the same household, like Ruby's. Such statistics do obscure heterogeneity within the suburbs themselves, and some children at Tūrama School are considerably better off than others. However, Tūrama School is overall designated as a "decile one, step A" school, indicating the highest of the eighteen levels of socioeconomic disadvantage used by the Ministry of Education to allocate funding.

Deprivation, in this context, manifests in some aspects of life more than others. Because state funding for Tūrama School is proportionally higher than funding for schools in more affluent areas, in some ways the children are quite well resourced. A cluster of around ten buildings, the school campus includes classroom blocks; an auditorium; several high-quality, safe playgrounds; sports fields; and a swimming pool. Tūrama School children's playtimes are enriched with play equipment, and they have access to information technologies in the classroom and library, high-quality teachers who care for and about them, smaller class sizes, and several field trips a year for education or celebration. For some children, school represents the warmest, healthiest, and safest environment they inhabit, although for many, the classroom comes with its own sets of social challenges. Many children come to school inadequately clothed and fed, and classrooms can be cold, leaky, or prone to flooding. Those who came to their end-of-year graduation prize-giving wore nice outfits, but half the graduating class were missing. Because parents often work multiple jobs with unconventional hours, their lack of availability means there are no school camps and no Saturday sports teams—both time-honored traditions of New Zealand school life. Tūrama School children may be developing their awareness of their inequitable circumstances, but their school experiences are still quite distinct from those at the decile ten school in the next district.

Tūrama School children are also not aware that in Aotearoa poverty has been found to increase the likelihood of a range of issues that impact children in the present and establish lifetime trajectories of disadvantage, including poor nutrition (Wham, Teh, Moyes, et al. 2015), health issues (Poulton, Caspi, Milne, et al. 2002), and educational achievement (Fergusson and Woodward 2000; Gibb, Fergusson, and Horwood 2012). Recent New Zealand research has demonstrated how the effects of poverty on brain development in the first few years of life can be carried throughout the life course. Results of the Dunedin longitudinal study show that around 20 percent of the population account for around 80 percent of adult economic burden, including 81 percent of criminal convictions, 66 percent of welfare benefits, 78 percent of prescription fills, and 40 percent of excess obese kilograms, and that these individuals, who were more likely to have grown up in socioeconomic deprivation or have experienced child maltreatment, could be reliably predicted *from neurological evaluation at age three* (Caspi, Houts, Belsky, et al. 2016). Poverty is also linked to child abuse, which remains a significant problem in New Zealand. The White Paper on Vulnerable Children reports that between seven and ten children are killed each year by a caregiver, while in the year leading up to June 2012, the organization responsible for care and protection issues, Child, Youth and Family (CYF, pronounced "sif" or "sifs"),[4] found 4,766 cases of neglect; 3,249 cases of physical abuse; 1,396 cases of sexual abuse; and 12,114 cases of emotional abuse (often involving children witnessing family violence) (Ministry of Social Development 2012). Internationally, childhood abuse, along with other adverse childhood experiences including the loss, incarceration, mental illness, or drug or alcohol abuse of a parent, has been linked to a range of health conditions later in life including obesity, cancer, addiction, diabetes, and stroke (Bynum, Griffin, Riding, et al. 2010; Felitti, Anda, Nordenberg, et al. 1998; Gilbert, Breiding, Merrick, et al. 2015).

These socioeconomic pressures therefore have significant impact over the life course, and they create particular experiences of childhood. For Tūrama School children, their relative deprivation is mostly unseen, except perhaps when they attend an interschool *kapa haka*[5] competition and notice the clean and fancy uniforms of the largely Pākehā private school children also in attendance. This could be quite a different experience for socioeconomically deprived children attending a high decile school. Yet Tūrama School children do notice who is requesting a stigmatized "spare lunch," they manage their cold and sick bodies, and they are devastated by the poverty-related illness or death of family members. For many, family violence, or "getting a hiding," is a normal part of life, but the threat of being "taken away" by CYF means children will also work to conceal specific violent events from teachers.

These are the *practices* of children negotiating the structuring conditions of their lives: making meanings from material deprivation that in turn become the webs that govern their sociality; making accommodations in some domains to compensate for deprivation in others; caring for their health in the face of epidemic disease. The reasons for these circumstances, however, go much deeper, arising as a consequence of their colonization and migration histories. In the following two sections, I outline the respective histories of these relationships with specific reference to Papakura and the health outcomes that disproportionately affect Māori and Pasifika children in this region.

Colonial Legacies and Health

The demographic pattern of Tūrama School, which shapes their views of the country, identities, and peer relations, has long historical roots that privilege Pākehā over Māori and other ethnic groups and that contribute to current health disparities in Papakura as well as nationally. The early colonial history of the Papakura region is well documented in several volumes (Craig 1982; Smith 2016) and by the Papakura Museum from archival material. I spent several hours in this museum building a picture of the events that have led to the current circumstances of Tūrama School children.

Postcolonial New Zealand history is built around an often fraught relationship between Māori and Pākehā, which, since the signing of the Treaty of Waitangi in 1840, has seen Māori stripped of their lands, language, and culture and marginalized, and which has set in motion cycles of intergenerational trauma that play out for the children of Tūrama School to this day (Pihama, Reynolds, Smith, et al. 2014; Wirihana and Smith 2014). Craig (1982) details how the events following the treaty established the Pākehā stronghold in the Papakura region. Prior to the treaty, the South Auckland (Manukau) region appears to have been sparsely populated by Māori, who roamed the wider area and resided seasonally in the Papakura area, taking advantage of a rich food bowl and cultivating some gardens. In the early 1840s, three European families established a settlement in Papakura and built what accounts suggest seem to have been friendly relationships with local Māori, sharing agricultural practices, and settler children growing up speaking Te Reo (the Māori language) alongside their Māori playmates. This relationship became strained in the early 1860s. Under the Treaty, the crown had reserved a pre-emptive right to purchase Māori lands, and in 1853 the governor, facing increased demand for land by settlers, reduced the price per acre, which saw an erosion of Māori holdings as the land was snapped up by wealthy speculators.

The colonial government then prepared to invade the Waikato region in 1863 to claim Māori land under the pretense of forcing the allegiance of local iwi to the Crown (Sinclair 2000). As the gateway to the Waikato region, Papakura was designated as a place of strategic importance, and a large military road was built connecting the two regions, which local Māori viewed with unease and protested. The tensions resulted in many Māori leaving the area to seek refuge in Waikato, while others were labeled as rebels and forced to leave the district. Large blocks of Māori-owned land, including villages and sacred places, were then confiscated by the government, justified as punishment for a rebellion that had not eventuated. This land was parceled up and distributed for settlement to military men who had fought in the Land Wars and new European migrants arriving under the 1864 Waikato Immigration Scheme to settle the frontier between Auckland and Waikato. From 1865 the Māori population of Papakura was all but eliminated, while descendants of the European settler families who developed the region into a thriving business center remain in Papakura to this day.

The return of Māori to Papakura is less clearly documented, but from the late 1930s, population growth and the advent of World War II opened up new opportunities for urban employment and resulted in a mass migration of Māori to urban centers. Between 1936 and 1986, an 83 percent rural Māori population became an 83 percent urban population (Belich 2001), many of whom tended to have less education and who, away from traditional whānau and hapū connections, struggled with poverty. Māori-run organizations such as the Māori Women's Welfare League were set up to meet the needs of urban-based Māori, including housing and pastoral care (Hill 2009, as cited in Gagné 2013). While the Māori cultural renaissance of the 1970s and 1980s saw the establishment of new *marae*[6] in Auckland and the revival of Te Reo and Māori activism, many urban Māori did not hold a strong sense of Māori identity (van Meijl 2006; Borrell 2005). State housing was built to accommodate many of these Māori throughout Auckland. Meanwhile, Papakura saw the establishment of a military base in 1939, which brought considerable wealth and prestige to the area. The military base was closed in 1992, and the land was carved up for new developments, including state housing. In 2000, Papakura was again one of several areas of "high deprivation" in South Auckland targeted for new state housing that became home to low-income Māori as well as Pacific migrants. The families of Māori children at Tūrama School, therefore, are from various iwi, and many maintain ties to marae in Northland, Waikato, or the rural east. Others have connections to the Papakura marae, which was established in 1979 to serve the wider community while acknowledging Waikato-Tainui and Ngati Tamaoho as *tangata whenua* (original inhabitants). Others still have little or no connection to Māori culture, may not know their iwi, and do not identify with a marae.

The impacts of colonization have been desolating for Māori, who are disproportionately represented in statistics for almost every major indicator of health and well-being, from mortality and hospitalization rates (well summarized by Reid, Taylor-Moore, and Varona 2014) to educational achievement (Marie, Fergusson, and Boden 2008). It should be noted that such statistics conceal the wide variation in circumstances across Māori from the top to the bottom of the socioeconomic ladder (Durie 2001); the group of children I worked with at Tūrama School are not *representative* of Māori but instead are among the most disadvantaged of Māori. However, these disparities can be consistently traced upstream not only to socioeconomic disadvantage but also the intergenerational transmission of the historical trauma of colonization, the collective disenfranchised grief, stress, and dislocation from culture that have destabilized the *wairua* (spirit) of whānau and iwi (Pihama, Reynolds, Smith, et al. 2014; Wirihana and Smith 2014; Reid, Varona, Fisher, et al. 2016). These traumas are perpetuated through health care and education that is still, for the most part, delivered through colonizing institutions. Māori also experience higher levels of racial discrimination, which has documented negative effects on health and achievement (Blank, Houkamau, and Kingi 2016; Harris, Tobias, Jeffreys, et al. 2006; Harris, Cormack, and Stanley 2013; Turner, Rubie-Davies, and Webber 2015). For the children I worked with, some steps have been taken to correct this problem, with a bilingual unit that operates semi-autonomously in Tūrama School according to Māori *tikanga* (customs), and through marae-based services such as those offered by the Papakura marae, which include food parcels and community meals, justice programs, a primary care clinic, and a pharmacy service. The marae also coordinates the Manakidz throat-swabbing program that operates at Tūrama School. New Zealand still has far to go before the damage may begin to be reversed, however, and the consequences of this colonial legacy can be seen in the health status of Tūrama School children—in particular, the rheumatic fever that caused Victor's leaky heart valve.

Pasifika Migration Histories

Pasifika families in New Zealand, too, disproportionately share these strained socioeconomic circumstances and subsequent impacts on health. Most of the 20 percent of children at Tūrama School who are Pasifika identify as Tongan or Samoan and were born in Auckland, although some are recent migrants. While historical processes of colonization underlie the material disadvantage of Māori children, the inequitable living circumstances of Pasifika children stem from Tongan and Samoan migration histories. Large-scale migration from Polynesia to Aotearoa began after World War II, when migrants were encouraged as workers to help with labor-shortages in a booming economy. People from Tokelau, Niue, and Cook Islands were deemed to be New Zealand citizens, while migrants from Western Samoa and Tonga were required to apply for a work permit, although the practice of "turning a blind eye" to those working beyond their permit was commonplace as their labor was in demand (Savelio 2005).

From the mid-1970s, an economic downturn particularly affected manufacturing industries in which many Pasifika were engaged and left communities struggling with high levels of unemployment. Societally, Pasifika peoples were cast as a threat to New Zealand and blamed for problems with law and order (Dunsford, Park, Littleton, et al. 2011). From 1974, "dawn raids" were made on the homes of alleged overstayers, and even some individuals with valid work permits were forcibly repatriated (Macpherson 1996; Liava'a 1998). These raids, often carried out at dawn to catch women and children while male family members worked the night shift, created a climate of fear and made "Islanders" the targets of antagonism, stigmatization, and discrimination.

By 1991, the number of "Pacific" people born in New Zealand equaled the number of migrants, and success in sports, arts, and community work, including high-profile festivals, improved perceptions of Pasifika peoples (Dunsford, Park, Littleton, et al. 2011). However, as a result of barriers including language, education, and discrimination, Pasifika migrants and descendants are still often relegated into low-paying labor or shift work and low-cost, poor-quality rental housing, which adds stress for families. Throughout the migration period until the present, Pasifika peoples have struggled with housing, because of discrimination by landlords and the prohibitive cost of renting or buying homes in Auckland. The radical policies of economic deregulation and liberalization of the early 1990s led to a restructuring of social welfare and corporatization of state-housing programs, including adoption of "market rates" by Housing New Zealand, which caused rents for low-income tenants to rise by 106 percent from 1992 to 1999, compared with a 23 percent increase in the private rental sector (Cheer, Kearns, and Murphy 2002). Consequently, housing-related poverty became more widespread through the 1990s (Thorns 2000) and families often "doubled up" to save costs (Howden-Chapman, Pene, Crane, et al. 2000), filling garages, sheds, and caravans, and in damp, uninsulated accommodations. As the government sold state-owned housing in gentrified, middle-class neighborhoods, rising rents saw the increased relocation of Pasifika peoples—along with Māori—to outer, southern and western suburbs of Auckland (Dunsford, Park, Littleton, et al. 2011), including Papakura.

Pasifika have also seen a shift in patterns of disease over the migration history, with the rise of noncommunicable diseases such as diabetes and heart disease, along with lingering communicable diseases such as tuberculosis. For children, disparities in health measures between Pasifika and non-Pasifika in Aotearoa have been apparent since systematic tracking of Pasifika children began in the 1970s (Dunsford, Park, Littleton, et al. 2011), including obesity (Anderson, Gorman, and Lines 1977; Bell and Parnell 1996); nutritional deficiencies (Bell and Parnell 1996; Wilson, Grant, and Wall 1999); asthma (Ellison-Loschmann, Pattemore, Asher, et al. 2009; Mitchell and Cutler 1984); and communicable diseases including measles (Hardy, Lennon, and Mitchell 1987; Steele 1973) meningococcal A and B (Baker, McNicholas, Garrett, et al. 2000; Lennon, Gellin, Hood, et al. 1993; Wilson, Baker, Martin, et al. 1995), and respiratory illness (Grant 1999). Of particular interest to this book, disparities for rheumatic fever have been recorded since the 1980s, and from 1980 to 1984 the rate for Pasifika children under fifteen years old was between nine and ten times the rate for European children (Lennon, Martin, Wong, et al. 1988). This discrepancy has continued to this day; in 2016, after four years of intervention programs, rheumatic fever rates for Pasifika children are still nearly four times higher than for Māori and eight times higher than the national rate (Ministry of Health 2017). For many schools in socioeconomically disadvantaged areas of the country, efforts to combat rheumatic fever have become a prominent feature of school life, meaning that even though only a handful of children at the school would ever develop the disease, it has become significant to the coproduction of health for every child at Tūrama School.

Rheumatic Fever

Among the confluence of physical and social disruptions that have marked Victor's body, it is the heart valve damage following rheumatic fever that has attracted recent government attention and intervention on a national scale. An autoimmune response to group A streptococcus (GAS) infection, acute rheumatic fever is a major cause of childhood morbidity and mortality in mainly developing countries (Carapetis, Steer, Mulholland, et al. 2005). Rheumatic fever occurs mainly in children aged five through fourteen, with mean incidence in New Zealand peaking at ages nine through twelve (Milne, Lennon, Stewart, et al. 2012).

The chief concern with rheumatic fever is the inflammation of the heart (carditis), which can cause damage to the cardiac valve, or "heart damage" as it is described in lay terms (Jaine, Baker, and Venugopal 2008), and can lead to chronic rheumatic heart disease (CRHD) in later life (Milne, Lennon, Stewart, et al. 2012). While rheumatic fever is rarely fatal for New Zealand children, the CRHD that often follows is a significant cause of premature death in Aotearoa, and the state's failure to prevent rheumatic fever now means a burden for decades to come for those communities worst affected (Wilson 2010). The experience of a common childhood GAS infection—strep throat—can therefore result in a sequelae of subsequent illnesses for the rest of an individual's life.

Rates of rheumatic fever, a disease associated with developing countries, increased in New Zealand by 59 percent between 1993 and 2009 (Milne, Lennon, Stewart, et al. 2012), driven almost exclusively by rising incidences for Māori and Pasifika children (Jaine, Baker, and Venugopal 2008). The discrepancy is startling; mean incidence rates between 2000 and 2009 were 81.2 (per 100,000) for Pasifika children and 40.2 for Māori children, compared to just 2.1 for non-Māori/ Pasifika (predominantly Pākehā) children. A 2012 epidemiological study found that while Māori and Pacific children constituted 30 percent of children in the 2006 census, they accounted for 92 percent of new cases of rheumatic fever in the period between 2000 and 2009 (Milne, Lennon, Stewart, et al. 2012). Although twin studies indicate a genetic susceptibility to rheumatic fever exists at an individual level, there is no evidence that these ethnic disparities reflect population-level genetic differences (Bryant, Robins-Browne, Carapetis, et al. 2009; Carapetis, Currie, and Mathews 2000). Even in populations heavily exposed to GAS bacteria, no more than around 3 to 6 percent of children are expected to develop rheumatic fever (Carapetis, Currie, and Mathews 2000).

The overrepresentation of Māori and Pasifika children in New Zealand's rheumatic fever statistics is therefore the result of a complex interplay between biological and socially mediated factors: individual susceptibility and GAS virulence, and levels of bacteria exposure and treatment with antibiotics (Carapetis, Currie, and Mathews 2000). These factors appear to be influenced by socioeconomic disadvantage (household overcrowding, increased incidence of streptococcal upper respiratory tract infections, decreased health-care access) (Jaine, Baker, and Venugopal 2011; Milne, Lennon, Stewart, et al. 2012; Wilson 2010). A recent epidemiological study in New Zealand demonstrated a steep increase in incidence rates for rheumatic fever with degree of socioeconomic deprivation (Milne, Lennon, Stewart, et al. 2012), with the highest deprivation quintile accounting for 70 percent of hospital admissions among children aged five to fourteen. The cumulative risk for a child living in a region of high socioeconomic disadvantage—like the area where Tūrama School is located—is 0.0066, about a 1-in-150 risk of being admitted to hospital for rheumatic fever (Milne, Lennon, Stewart, et al. 2012). At Tūrama School, this child is Victor.

The experience of rheumatic fever for children like Victor begins with a lengthy hospital stay followed by ten years of monthly prophylactic penicillin injections to prevent secondary recurrences. Victor, like most children, receives his injection at school, where the district nurse comes by to administer the injection to him and several others. However, after incidence rates in these socioeconomically disadvantaged groups rose above a threshold of more than fifty per 100,000 children, attention shifted to primary prevention. In 2011, the New Zealand government established the Rheumatic Fever Prevention Programme (RFPP) with the aim of reducing rheumatic fever admissions by two-thirds (Ministry of Health 2013). The major component of the RFPP targets GAS bacteria, with funding allocated for free throat swabs for high-risk groups at primary care rapid-response clinics and free clinics in schools in areas of high economic deprivation. A secondary component involves health promotion to families and health professionals. Least emphasis is put on the third aspect: strategies to address social and environmental factors such as poor housing and household crowding. Funding is also allocated for research, surveillance, and primary care development.

Thus, the disease that has shaped Victor's childhood is now structurally integrated into the lives of all children at Tūrama School through their "sore throat clinic," which links Victor to children like Dante, who visits the school clinic almost weekly to have his throat checked, and Teuila, who diligently takes her antibiotics only every second day so that her siblings might have the other half, and Marielle, who tells her friends she has rheumatic fever, not realizing her diagnosis is actually for strep throat. While the clinical and political implications of rheumatic fever policy are to greater and lesser degrees the subject of policy attention, what lies underneath is the power of the clinic to *infiltrate*, just as it is *infiltrated by* the institutional activities that bring it to life in situ. The clinic becomes woven into classroom dynamics while simultaneously restructuring the school day; the clinic is both synthesized into new productions of knowledge and reconfigures children's relationships to their bodies. Chapters 4 and 6 describe the processes through which this occurs, as underpinned by the roles of the state and the institution in child health detailed in the next section.

State and Institutional Roles in Health

Ruby had been experiencing stomach pains for several days but remained at school while the office and her teacher, Mrs. Randall, tried unsuccessfully to contact her mother. "You need to tell your mum to take you to the doctor," Mrs. Randall told her, stern with worry, as Ruby curled up against me, hot and listless. The next day Ruby did not come to school, but she was back the day after, swinging on her chair. "Are you feeling better?" I asked, and she nodded.

"Not really," said Mrs. Randall, speaking for Ruby. Later that day, she tells me she'd asked Ruby whether she went to a doctor. "She said she had," said Mrs. Randall, "and I asked her what the doctor said, and she said the doctor said she had a sore stomach. So I asked if the doctor had checked for appendicitis and she said yes. But I don't think she went to the doctor at all." Mrs. Randall thought Ruby was covering for her parents. The family had access to a doctor at the marae, so Mrs. Randall reckoned Ruby's parents "couldn't be bothered" taking her. "But I will keep calling them and telling them she needs to go," Mrs. Randall concluded.

Much responsibility for managing the problem of children in poverty ultimately falls on New Zealand schools, but the multiple roles played by the institution in caring for children's health and well-being sit in tension with neoliberal discourses that frame child poverty as a problem of parental responsibility. Situated as it is in an economically deprived area, Tūrama School participates in an especially large number of such initiatives, supported by national or local government or nongovernmental organizations (NGOs), for the purpose of caring for children's bodies. At the time of my fieldwork, these included government-funded services (the dental service, fruit in schools, throat and skin checks, social workers in schools); corporate-sponsored services (milk in schools; school provided services: basic first aid, some provision of school uniform, spare lunches, sports equipment and lunch time sports games); and NGO-sponsored services (head lice checks and treatment; breakfast in schools; visits from the Life Education bus; provision of jackets, shoes, and basic hygiene supplies such as tissues and hand sanitizer). The school itself supports all of these initiatives with class time, organization, distribution, and administration. As well as these formal initiatives, the school has an informal role in looking after children's bodies, and teachers and other staff regularly diagnose and make decisions on children's ailments and actively educate about or promote healthy behaviors. There are also external services, such as CYF, which often operate through the school.

For Tūrama School, this creates an environment where teachers grapple with the boundaries of their role, alternately motivated by a desire to "make a difference" and frustrated and fatigued by the demands of caring for twenty-odd children while under Ministry of Education pressure to improve student performance on the national standardized tests. Teachers generally made their own decisions about what role to play, and so Mrs. Charles gave Ruby and other pupils her phone number and picked up Mila one night from the train station in the next district after she ran away from home. Mrs. Randall intervened to make sure Ruby saw a doctor and used her own money to buy stationery for one girl and a swimsuit for another so that she could join the class in the pool. Mrs. Stevens, who drives one boy to school every day to ensure he actually attends, reflected that while these things should be the parent's responsibility, in her view, schools had to be "realistic"; for instance, when parents are not taking children to a doctor, the school needs to step in. "Shouldn't have to, but I think they do have to," she concluded.

This conclusion—"We *shouldn't* have to but we *do* have to"—and the accompanying fatigue and resentment are shared by many of the staff and cause great internal conflict. A senior staff member, frustrated by the intrusion of health and NGO services into education, sums up, and then immediately criticizes his own position: "Me, I would say no milk, no fruit, no free jackets, no shoes, which is probably not a very good decision."

The role of state schools in child health is not new, but understandings of the role have shifted and, to a large extent, become more ambiguous under neoliberalism. Aotearoa has an established history of embracing a "welfare state" for population health and well-being and with particular concern for children. The first decades of the twentieth century saw an emerging interest of central government in child health and welfare, beginning with a raft of policies legislating for lower income tax for families with dependents (1914), a minimum-wage calculated for the support of children (1920), and a benefit for families with more than two children (1927) (Easton 1980). The welfare state was entrenched in the 1938 Social Security Act, which encompassed a range of material benefits for the protection of particular groups, including widows, the disabled, and the elderly, followed by the 1946 universal family benefit and the domestic purposes benefit for single parents in 1973. Throughout this time, schools have functioned as key sites of state health surveillance and intervention (Burrows and

Wright 2007; Kearns and Collins 2000). From as early as 1920, school dental clinics were established to supply free dental treatment to all children until age eighteen (Saunders 1964), while health and hygiene was a key concern of early New Zealand industrial schools for homeless or delinquent children (Matthews 2000). By the late 1940s, all children underwent routinized medical examinations at school, and those who were not "thriving" in their home environment were sent to state-sponsored "health" camps (Kearns and Collins 2000), some of which persist today, although there are far fewer and they cater to a much narrower group of children. Aspects of state care continue in the present, including publicly funded health services and a 2004 Working for Families benefit that supplements the incomes of working parents (Taxation [Working for Families] Act 2004).

However, the 1980s and 1990s saw dramatic shifts in economic policy and state welfare, the effects of which on low-income populations are still felt to this day (Poata-Smith 2013). The once-popular ethos of the welfare state eroded from the mid-1970s as economic and political changes led to rising inflation, public debt, and unemployment. In 1984 the Labour government adopted the economic policies of the early 1980s United Kingdom and United States, known as "neoliberalism," to dramatically restructure state functioning in accordance with competitive market principles: opening up the economy to international markets and corporatizing and privatizing state-owned commercial operations and assets (Larner 1997). The effect of these was a further rise in unemployment, peaking in 1991. This peak coincided with the introduction of major welfare reforms by the new National government, which slashed benefits; restructured state housing provisions to require profit; and introduced employment law reform to deregulate the labor market, remove protections for workers, and undermine collective wage bargaining (Larner 1997; Nairn, Higgins, and Sligo 2012). The subsequent rise in poverty disproportionately impacted Māori and Pasifika families, who were more likely to be employed in low-wage manufacturing or to be on benefits (welfare), and particularly impacted children, of whom 29 percent were in the lowest income quintile (Atwool 1999; Poata-Smith 2013). By 1998, social policy initiatives were being discursively framed in terms of "social responsibility," materializing in the distribution throughout the New Zealand population of a pamphlet entitled *Towards a Code of Social and Family Responsibility: Public Discussion Document*, which stated an aim of clarifying the responsibilities of families, particularly parents, in order to reduce government spending (Larner 2000; Tap 2007). Further welfare reforms in 1998, 2006, and 2013 continued to tighten the criteria for receiving a benefit and reconfigured welfare payments in terms of employment-seeking support (Social Security Act 1964). Heavy penalties for not meeting benefit criteria were reported to have cut payments for 43,000 parents in the two years following the 2012 reform, alarming child welfare interest groups (Migone 2015).

The rise of neoliberalism also saw a withdrawal of central government from schools and a reframing of schools as "self-managing" under a 1989 reform (Wylie 1994). The idea was to move away from a one-size-fits-all approach to child health and hand over the power and decision-making process to local communities to decide what their priorities are and what approach is most useful. Although Sinkinson (2011) notes that educating individuals to be accountable for their own health status has been an enduring aspect of the curriculum since the early twentieth century; at the same time, neoliberal ideologies infused schools with "healthism," discourses of health based on an ideology of individualism and pre-supposing that individuals should take responsibility for their own health status. For example, as part of the "Health Promoting Schools" movement initiated by the World Health Organization, the 2005 Fruit in Schools program gave a free piece of fruit to each child in low-decile schools, but it came tagged with an educational mandate to "promote healthy lifestyles" and approaches that "empowered" students with the responsibility for educating their peers and creating health-promoting programs and environments (Boyd 2011). However, in localizing the solutions, the state also localizes responsibility for the problems—problems that in many cases are produced by structural conditions much greater than the local community. Children's dietary habits are constrained by the affordability of fruit, itself governed by national and global markets, seasonal climates, pests, and pathogens, as well as national-level policy factors, including tightened restrictions on access to benefits; increasing rents from a housing shortage in Auckland city; a low minimum-wage level; and epidemics of addiction, domestic violence, and mental illness (Reid, Taylor-Moore, and Varona 2014). While Tūrama School children largely conceptualized health in terms of eating fruit and vegetables, for many, the government provisions were the *only* fruit they could eat that week. The intent to establish responsibility for healthy eating without changing the constraining conditions means that while technically a Health Promoting School, Tūrama School has not followed the criteria for the last few years, and the only aspect of the Fruit in Schools program remaining is the free fruit.

The economic and housing insecurity wrought by neoliberalism also contribute to high rates of transience as families move when rents rise or children are passed between kin. Polynesian childhoods are embedded in the wider family, whether that be the Māori whānau, the Samoan *aiga*, or the Tongan *kainga*, and within this fluid kinship, adult kin other than parents are typically seen as equally influential in the support and guidance of children (Brady 1976; Carroll 1970; Metge 1995; Morton 1996; Ritchie and Ritchie 1979). Widespread across Polynesia are *whāngai* practices, which loosely entail adoption (but not in the formal or legal sense of the English word), with children being placed with kin other than biological parents for reasons such as continuing a family name, strengthening whānau bonds, or alleviating financial pressure. Although the introduction of the Domestic Purposes Benefit in 1973 meant that single mothers could now care for their children themselves (Metge 1995), in the present day, children can still commonly be "whāngai-ed" out to other relatives, particularly grandparents, in the short or long term when circumstances—especially economic and housing instability—necessitate (Gagné 2013). Thus, Ruby's youngest brother is also her auntie's son, and both of them live in Ruby's household. Often, when children are in situations of abuse or neglect, whānau members, particularly *kaumātua* (elders), may intervene and negotiate for the child to stay with another whānau member. Hence nine-year-old Whetu lived with his grandmother for several years, and ten-year-old Cassidee and eleven-year-old Trystan lived with their respective aunties.

Whāngai practices are not recognized under New Zealand law, however, and this privileging of Western colonial family structures has had harrowing impacts for Māori. Following a number of high-profile journalistic reports (e.g. Forbes, 2017), an independent inquiry was initiated in 2018 to investigate the disproportionate numbers of Māori children who were "uplifted" (CYF terminology) from whānau since the mid-twentieth century and placed under state care, where many were physically, sexually, or psychologically abused. While best practice now involves working with whānau, hapū, and iwi in the uplifting and appropriate placement of Māori children, this is not always accomplished, and certainly the historical trauma of whānau disruptions by the state have had long-lasting, intergenerational effects for whānau in the present.[7]

Many Tūrama School children therefore move back and forth between places of care, often changing schools as well. New Zealand family policy and education systems, however, are based on Western beliefs and values, including an assumption that the nuclear family is the main and superior unit of social organization (Durie-Hall and Metge 1992; Metge 1995; Morehu 2005; Ritchie and Ritchie 1979, 1997). This means that the basic design of policies for housing, health, employment, education and social services, as well as legal concepts of adoption, guardianship, and parental rights, have not always effectively taken into account the cultural needs of the people who could most benefit from the support. One way in which this issue impacts children is that the institution-based education systems are designed for stable, nuclear families and do not accommodate the transience of whānau or the many children who "boomerang" (Gilbert 2005, viii) in and out of schools like Tūrama School over the year. For children, as I discuss in chapter 7, shifting schools during the school year can mean disrupted peer and teacher relationships and impacted academic progress (Gilbert 2005; Mutch, Rarere, and Stratford 2011; Wynd 2014), while the social instability that this transience creates has important implications for health.

Children's health, therefore, is profoundly shaped by the realization of neoliberal ideologies through the school institution: in the formal interventions that offer throat checks and free fruit; in the way that teachers balance finding the boundaries of their role with their own affective sense of care; or in the multiple transitions that pupils must make from one institution to another. But children do not passively experience the impacts of these structures on their health; they actively meet, negotiate, and transform them. What remains missing from this picture is what I have alluded to throughout this chapter: the experiences, understandings, and collective meanings and practices of children themselves that contribute to the coproduction of these environments, the children's bodies, and their health. The remainder of this book will therefore forefront children's perspectives of living and practicing these Aotearoa childhoods.

3

Negotiating Generational Differences in Ethical Research

Two interacting but distinct worlds coexist within Tūrama School; the sparsely populated but hierarchically privileged adult world, and the populous but subordinate world of children. These worlds are maintained by separate sets of written and unwritten rules for staff and students in the school, but also the organization and daily practices of members of both. Space that appears to be shared is in fact fractured with tiny implicit boundaries demarcating who goes into which place and what they do there. In the classroom, children occupy small desks accompanied by small chairs, and sit or lie on the mat, while teachers have big desks and sit on big chairs at the edges of children's space. Elsewhere, adults congregate in staff-only spaces and offices and the tea room, while children requesting help or delivering a message will stand with their toes in line with the door frames, cautiously peering in, waiting to catch the attention of an adult occupant. Children's habitats are found in the familiarity of the playgrounds, sports fields, and school library, while teachers patrol the peripheries in fluorescent safety vests. In assemblies, children sit in rows on the hard auditorium floor, surveyed by teachers who sit at the end. Their spaces are further partitioned by age and gender, and these are maintained by children themselves; seniors guide wayward juniors back over the line painted through the middle of the hot asphalt courts while shrieks caution boys to steer clear of the girls' bathrooms. The school is patterned by invisible stripes and spots, zoned by identity and status, marked by boundaries that are not seen but *felt*, the sense of exposure as eyes are drawn to a body that is disproportionate to those around it, out of place. This architectural and physical segregation of the child and adult populations is what Foucault (1979) identifies as a mechanism of power that works to enable access to the bodies, actions, and attitudes of individuals. Adults hold absolute authority here, but not absolute power, as children adapt to, ignore, resist, or internalize power structures in their own quiet or unquiet way.

The school's architectural ordering, temporal organization by age group and time of day and season, and governing rules and systems are adult creations to maintain adult authority (Foucault 1979). Within this space however, to use Corsaro's analogy, children work like spiders, spinning webs of meaning across everything they find (Corsaro 2015). These webs are largely disregarded by adults, if they are seen at all, and coming to understand children's cultures, without disrupting, misrepresenting, or colonizing them has been a problem of adult researchers for more than three decades. In this chapter I consider one aspect of this problem: the issue of navigating generational differences in fieldwork. Although focusing on research ethics, this chapter also foregrounds the relational in producing the knowledge that supports this book, and thus sets out the epistemology of what is to come.

It was into this highly segregated world that I arrived, an adult most similar not only generationally but ethnically and socioeconomically to the authoritative adults, rather than the children from whom I wanted to learn.[1] Anthropologists and sociologists (Christensen 2004; Fine and Sandstrom 1988; James 2001; Mandell 1988; Mayall 2000) have long remarked on the role of the researcher as a central and uniquely challenging issue in studies with children, and this is particularly the case in institutional settings such as schools where differences in status and authority are most systematically, ritually, and symbolically drawn and maintained. In anthropology the role of the researcher—or who the researcher is in relation to others in the field—has been vigorously debated with regard to adults (Adler and Adler 1987; Gold 1958), particularly with the rise of engaged or activist anthropology (Scheper-Hughes 1995), and is certainly also a source of ethical or practical tension in adult research (Kloos 1969). However, the relations of authority embedded in child and adult bodies create particular problems in fieldwork with children. For studies in which children are accompanied by adults, it is almost inevitable that adult concerns are asserted. Moreover, subgroups such as parents and teachers both hold authority over the children who are the focus of research and act as gatekeepers regulating researcher access and child participation. Finally, in traditional ethnographic settings researchers tend to assume an equal status with their research subjects— or at least assume that participants should be treated as equals. Fine and Sandstrom (1988), however, argue that child research is distinct even from research with other protected groups such as the mentally disabled, because the social code requires that legitimate adult-child relationships be governed by adult authority.

Nevertheless, the focus of ethical guidelines for children tends to be on entry to the field and discrete ethical moments (Christensen and Prout 2002)—consent, confidentiality, protection from harm—rather than on the ongoing, performative practice of intersubjectivity that constitutes fieldwork (Meloni, Vanthuyne, and Rousseau 2015; Shore and Trnka 2013). For adult researchers working with children, bypassing the authority structures embedded in generational relations without undermining them, and navigating the expectations of other adults while maintaining allegiance to child participants, constitute an often impossible task. This is a particular problem with participant observation, in which the researcher hopes to integrate into a natural setting and must work within established power structures, in contrast to interviews, focus groups, or workshops, which are already marked as out-of-the-ordinary events and may be constituted within a special set of rules.

With all these complications, how then are adult researchers to approach participant observation in schools? In this chapter I consider this question in reference to popular suggested researcher roles, namely the "friend" (Fine and Sandstrom 1988), the "least adult" (Mandell 1988), and the "unusual" or "different sort of adult" (Christensen 2004). Although psychological paradigms have tended toward more detached observational roles, the social sciences have been concerned with understanding data as produced through relationships; hence researchers such as Mandell (1988), Mayall (2000), and Christensen (2004) seek roles that explicitly avoid authority but facilitate acceptance by children as participants in their social interactions. While these researchers acknowledge that there is no one ideal role of the adult researcher, nor is any role free from tensions and dilemmas, I discuss two specific problems I encountered within my "different kind of adult" role. First, there can often be a discrepancy between how adults expect or perceive children to be and how children actually are. Researchers who are granted access to children's worlds can become mired in political "stickiness" when confronted with children's taboo behaviors, caught between conflicting ethical and cultural values. Second, children rely on known categories of adult "type" in order to successfully navigate the political quagmire that is being a child in an adult-dominated institution. While I was concerned with building rapport, in trying to distance myself from adult authority the ambiguity of my role from children's perspectives created the conditions for disclosures that required me to break confidentiality, with significant impact for participants.

I therefore highlight the importance of relational perspectives on researcher roles, including the perspectives of adult and child participants who must read and interpret this role in the context of their daily lives. To navigate the tensions that can arise from intergenerational fieldwork, I propose the "transparent guest" as an operational mode for fieldwork. Although similar to the "different kind of adult" role, the transparent guest has two main features that help to demystify how intergenerational structures and rules are negotiated. First, most children have either hosted or themselves been a "guest," and understand that guests can bring with them rules from home that are different to those in the host environment. The role of guest therefore establishes the researcher as someone governed by a set of rules different from those for either adults or children in the school. Second, a policy of transparency, of naming what the researcher can or cannot do and why, makes those rules visible to children and other adults in the institution and can help to minimize issues arising from unknown or unpredictable codes of behavior. Researchers may then also deal with politically sticky situations by enlisting the help of children sympathetic to the worry of breaking a rule or getting into trouble. Importantly, both of these aspects form part of an ongoing relational and co-constructed process of negotiating how researchers and participants can be with one another.

Roles of the Adult Fieldworker in Research with Children

Accompanying the burgeoning interest in child-centered research over the past three decades, the recognition that children have their own cultures (Corsaro 1979, 1992; Opie and Opie 1969), the turn toward research "with" rather than "on" children, and the children's-rights framework have all implicated the taken-for-granted role of adult researcher as critical to research ethics and validity. A number of researcher roles have been proposed in variable attempts to minimize or mitigate the power differences between child participants and adult researchers and to allow adults greatest access to children's private worlds while maintaining protections with what is seen as a uniquely vulnerable group. This is particularly a problem of the Western world, where children are cordoned off into separate, "child-friendly" spaces and there are few opportunities for children to interact with adults outside of the authority structures of parent-offspring and teacher-student (James and Prout 1990).

One solution has been to engage children as researchers, bypassing the problem of generational differences completely, or as research partners who facilitate the research process with their peers. This approach can, however, mean shifting the problem one step upstream, as researchers still need to negotiate their relationships with child partners. Others have argued that child-led research is not necessarily "better" or more ethical (Gallacher and Gallagher 2008), and certainly there are practical obstacles to child-led research. My own attempts to involve children as active partners were rather unsuccessful; I invited children to share their thoughts on my research questions or findings, but most children would shrug and say they didn't know. Realizing that a partnership would require giving children greater understanding of research purposes and methods, I began devising a set of workshops modeled after the child-led work coming from Children's Research Centre at the Open University (The Open University n.d.), with the idea of producing a book based on children's own ideas and experiences. In the end, this idea proved too ambitious for my limited resources and the institutional constraints of the school. Instead, I brought paper and pens to the outdoor table or to the library at lunchtime, and any child could come and draw with me. I did not tell them what to draw, but I said I was making a book about them and invited them to contribute by telling me what should be in the book or drawing a picture of either something they really liked to do or a time when things were difficult. Children also drew during interviews with me and in class time when they had finished their set tasks. In addition, I worked with small groups of children, recording their conversations about "what it is like to be a child." This was a topic they took to with gusto. While they drew, I compiled their thoughts and illustrations, along with some of my own, into a picture book on my laptop, adding photographic backgrounds and digitally coloring the pictures. Children would come, peer over my shoulder, and ask questions, but when I invited their thoughts they had little specific feedback, beyond nodding or saying it was cool. "We *do* do that," sometimes they would exclaim in surprise.

My attempts at explicit partnership, therefore, were rather unsuccessful, at least in part because, embedded as we were in everyday school contexts, mutuality could gain little traction when the institutionalized relational mode was hierarchical. Regardless, in many cases, adult researchers still wish to engage with child participants directly, and I do not think good research with children necessitates their partnership as coinvestigators. When working with children, then, what role should the researcher assume?

In her discussion of this question, Nancy Mandell (1988) classifies proposed researcher roles into discrete categories of participation level from detached observer to complete involvement. Alternatively, these roles can be seen as falling across a spectrum that reflects the degree to which researchers accept or reject the social implications of their own adultness (Table 1). At one end is what Mandell considers the essentializing position of deterministic fields such as developmental psychology, which hold that children's worlds are so distinct as to preclude adult participation of any sort, and the structure of age roles and adult ethnocentrism are immutable. At the other end, researchers such as Mandell (1988), Waksler (1986), and Goode (1986) contend that differences between adults and children are mostly ideological, and therefore all aspects of adultness except for physical size may be cast aside. Child researchers in social science tend to propose roles that fall between the middle and this latter end of the spectrum, including the role of "friend" (Fine and Sandstrom 1988), "least adult" (Mandell 1988), and "unusual adult" (Christensen 2004; Mayall 2000), all of which accept to some degree the identity of adult, but attempt to disrobe from the conventional authority and ethnocentrism usually associated with adults.

Towards the "rejecting adultness" end of the spectrum, Fine and Sandstrom (1988) propose viewing roles as functions of two axes, with the roles they identify—supervisor, leader, observer, and friend—representing four permutations of degree of authority and positive relation. The authors advocate the friend role as a semi-participatory approach, seeing its low authority and high positive relation as most conducive to ethical research. However, adult authority

TABLE 1

Spectrum of adult researcher roles, ranging from a view of adultness as immutable and precluding any access to children's cultures to an almost complete rejection of adultness apart from physical differences.

Adultness immutable ⟵————————————⟶ *Adultness rejected*

Adult researchers cannot access children's worlds	Adult researchers can access children's worlds as a different of unusual kind of adult	Adult researchers can access children's worlds as friends	Adult researchers can participate as children or "least adult" in children's worlds
Developmental psychology	Mayall (2000) Christensen (2004)	Fine and Sandstrum (1988)	Waksler (1986) Goode (1986) Mandell (1988)

is often not easily dismantled, and in many settings, such as institutions, researchers may be limited by the requirement of other adults that they align with more adult roles. The friend role also does not address the question of how generational differences may be approached, especially given the social illegitimacy of adult-child friendships in a culture in which the proper mode of adult-child relations involves the authoritative and responsible adult who protects and educates children.

Further still towards rejecting adultness, Mandell (1988) posits the "least adult" role, which, although criticized, still holds a great deal of influence (e.g., Randall 2012). The role involves full participation in children's activity in the "least adult manner possible." In her embodiment of this role in her fieldwork with two- and four-year-olds in two day care centers, Mandell initially observed, then imitated children's actions, oral expressions, and social exchanges, through trial and error coming to be, she claims, accepted as a kind of big child. By "following them into the sandbox" (1988, 45), Mandell became included in children's play and through experience learned the rituals and rules children create and use to govern their interactions. (Similar methodology was used to the same effect by Corsaro [1979], but Mandell takes this a step further from peripheral to full participation.) In attempting to minimize all difference between herself and the children, Mandell did not direct or correct children's actions, even participating in rule-breaking or rule-stretching on occasions, and avoided adult "helper" roles where possible.

Mandell's "least child" role has been critiqued by Mayall (2000) and Christensen (2004), both of whom arrived at an approach of "different" or "unusual kind of adult." This approach sees accepting the adultness of the researcher as important for understanding children's experiences, but attempts to create a new, different category of adult. While the "least child" approach attempts to show children that differences between adults and children can be diffused to near invisibility, Mayall argues that to children, a central characteristic of adults is that they have power over children. Good data on children's experience therefore cannot begin with downplaying that truth. Instead, Mayall's approach is to work with generational issues: "asking children directly, to help me, an adult, to understand childhood" (2000, 122). Through this approach, Mayall became recognized as a "non-official adult" in school settings, a person to whom children could complain about school, but still relate to as an adult. Moreover, in facilitating focus group conversations (an adult role) but unlike adults, sitting back from directing the discussion, Mayall was able to listen to the way that children used conversation to acquire—and produce—knowledge. By shifting her own behavior, Mayall found that children started to set aside the generational order and move out of "adult-question, child-reply mode" (2000, 126). Meanwhile, it was sometimes only through augmenting children's voices with parent and teacher accounts that Mayall could fully understand a child's experience.

Christensen (2004), meanwhile, criticizes the "least adult" role as idealistic "wishing away" of differences between children and adults. Like Mayall, her approach in fieldwork in a Danish school context was to embrace her status as adult, but consider with greater nuance the question of what is an adult, recognizing that when children ask the ubiquitous "Who are you?" they are engaging with wider notions of who we are to one another. What *kind* of adult the researcher embodies very much matters in determining the kind of relationships established, the kind of data that are elicited, and how ethically these interactions are navigated. Christensen's aim was not to assume the status of child but to walk a tightrope between being recognized as an "adult" while avoiding association with any known category of adult, and the accompanying preconceived ideas, practices and connotations associated with that category, as well as adulthood more generally. For example, while following some set "rules" for adults within the institution, Christensen would also follow children's "rules" and practices in participation with children—when joining or leaving a game—and avoid traditional adult roles such as correcting behavior, resolving disputes, or looking after children. As this "different sort of adult," Christensen did not attempt to minimize typical adult ways of relating to children, instead seeking to understand their views and wishes and treating these respectfully and as important.

Anthropological Perspectives on Researcher Roles

Writing from anthropology, Christensen brings a sense of ethics as an ongoing relational and performative process—something that can be missing from childhood studies in which ethical discussions tend to be grounded in universal definitions of childhood and children's rights (Meloni, Vanthuyne, and Rousseau 2015). However, it is this anthropological view of how generational differences are codified into modes of relations in the field that usefully illuminates implications of the researcher role. For example, teasing in the Tūrama School context is a common and usually benign relational mode between adults, but from adult to child can function as an assertion of power or socialization technique (Morton 1996) and between children represents a form of cruelty. Although teachers frequently teased children, the hurt looks when I tried gentle teasing (of children with whom I already had good relationships) told me that I needed to reflect more on how the implications of relational modes shifted with my positioning.

In this anthropological view of the ethical as relational, the role of the researcher becomes understood not as a predetermined, static set of rules that the researcher brings into the field, but as a plurality of relationships actively negotiated through everyday mundane interactions, dynamic and shifting, and working both ways, as the role of the researcher influences participants' modes of being, power relations, and ways of seeing themselves, and vice versa. The field is an ecology of dynamic relationships and interactions, which is altered without volition by the researcher's presence (Dominguez 2016). These characteristics are not unique to research with children but are foundational to unpacking the ways in which researchers play into or disrupt the generational power dynamics that are specific to child research. The researcher may reinforce or undermine the previous power structures, including teacher authority and also power dynamics within peer relations. The researcher brings new social capital that is disseminated in unequal ways and is used and manipulated by children and adults to reconfigure power dynamics. Other authors have noted the potential for children to take advantage of the researcher's privileges, and this was my experience as well— for example, when I was invited to play tennis, only to realize it was because the children had been told they were no longer allowed to borrow tennis balls, but I as an adult would be. At other times, it was the teachers who would use me to support their agenda, in strategies to shame or control students.

Thinking in relational terms also helps with integrating the "scientific and moral aspects of knowledge production," which Meskel and Pels (2005, 3) argue represents a more anthropological approach to ethics. In the postmodernist rethinking of epistemology as dialectical, knowledge itself is co-constructed through interactions; the research process is not so much *exposing* knowledge as *making* it (Clifford and Marcus 1986). This is a dynamic central to fieldwork, what John Borneman (2009) calls a "dialectical objectification," whereby through encounters, interlocutors make one another as subjects and objects, coproducing unique knowledges from the subsequent insights. Because of existing dynamics of authority between adults and children, however, adults may start overwriting children's knowledge; when I played back early interview recordings I noticed myself following up on what was important to me and missing what else was said, jumping into silences loaded with meaning, and interpreting children's utterances through my own adult lenses, without considering alternative ways of understanding. Furthermore, in a school context in which I was there as a classroom helper, I was very aware that I was shaping children's knowledge at the same time that I attempted to study it. A little way through the interview process I realized I was still trying to hold onto a purist concept of research and the researcher, attempting to elicit children's views without "tainting" them with my own perspectives. Yet knowledge is inextricably woven into relationships, produced and used through relationships, functioning as a commodity, capital, or as a gift, and especially intrinsic to adult-child relationships in which the control of knowledge works to maintain power dynamics (Foucault 1990). Slowly my interviews turned into dialogues with knowledge shared from both sides. The children seemed to value my explanations of antibiotic resistance and the knowledge that they had had strep throat, not rheumatic fever, and in turn their responses helped to clarify my knowledge of them. As much as I may try to represent what children know and how they know it, this representation cannot be parsed from *how I came to know* what they know and how I *contributed* to what they know. Ethical research, therefore, involves a process of paying attention to the *kinds* of understandings that are produced collaboratively within varying researcher-participant relationships—embedded within, rather than supplementary to knowledge production (Pels 2005). The picture book is a material product of this process, the knowledge within it a synthesis of their emic and my etic perspectives, and of the relationships I had with these children—including the fact that I held the greatest social as well as editorial power.

If ethical and scientific rigor are grounded in relationships, then this is where the kind of adult makes a difference. When Mayall was attending to rather than minimizing generational differences, she could focus on understanding how children work within the social order. When I took a more authoritative role—for example, when asked to be a leader of a group of children on a school trip—I experienced one side of childhood: the mode of relations with adult authority. I became the constraint they pushed against to run and shout and play, while I felt the dirty looks of museum staff. I learned a lot about how children relate to this kind of adult that day, as well as how museums are not designed for children. Other times I could be a "guest" child, joining in their games. When a group of girls invited me to participate in their lunchtime game involving rounds of questions, in sharing my own answers I learned about the girls' greatest fears, favorite movies, and crushes on boys. My adultness came back with a mention of my partner, and I then learned how the girls perceived the lives of women; they acted out a proposal and showered me with grass confetti. Attempting to shed adultness, as in the "least adult" role, therefore limits the knowledge produced, because it denies the realities of children's relationship to adults, the adult privilege the researcher holds and how children might be using it to their advantage, and the adult agendas the researchers bring with them that shape the choices being made—who the researcher follows and what the researcher notes down or remembers. Perhaps counterintuitively, in accepting adultness, the "unusual adult" role allows for greater attention to what kind(s) of adult the researcher embodies, using adult identity as an analytical lens for interpreting both researcher-participant relationships and the knowledge produced within them.

The "unusual adult" role is not without ethical problems, however. While all of the authors mentioned (particularly Mandell) acknowledge practical challenges in maintaining their roles within a field twisted with complex power dynamics and multidimensional practices, when I entered fieldwork at Tūrama School with the "different kind of adult" role in mind two problems emerged. First, setting aside conventional adult roles can become politically 'sticky" when researchers come across children's taboo behaviors, which would normally be policed by adults. Second, the ambiguity of a researcher role can mislead child participants. In the remainder of this chapter I detail how these two problems emerged to challenge my positioning in the field, and I propose the concept of "transparent guest" as an operational mode for negotiating such issues in fieldwork with children.

The Unsanctioned Activities of Childhood

The first problem arises with the discrepancy between how the adults in the field expect children to be and how children actually are. Authors have noted there is a darker side to children's private worlds that Western adults are not comfortable with, as this darker side does not fit within the neat construction of childhood as an innocent and "nice" world (James, Jenks, and Prout 1998; Christensen 1999). Accessing these areas of children's worlds can become wrought with political, social, and emotional tensions when researchers are seen by other adults as not acting as adults should—condoning or colluding with children's "inappropriate" behavior by failing to intervene or disavow the behavior, or by actually participating in the behavior.

Both Mandell (1988) and Christensen (1999) describe ethnographic moments of stumbling over children's practices that were unsanctioned by adults. In the day care center where Mandell conducted her research, urinating in the yard was a regular but forbidden practice. Mandell's solution, when children tried to involve her, was to leave the scene. Similarly, Christensen (1999) writes of her encounter during fieldwork at a Danish school with a group of ten-year-old boys who show her that they have taped up another boy, Danny, onto the floor of a cloakroom. She describes in detail the dynamics of the scenario: Danny struggling to free himself while smiling and laughing; the excited, but not aggressive demeanor of the other boys; the contrast between her confusion and unease and the relaxed and unaffected responses of the boys involved, including Danny himself. And she describes her internal conflict as an anthropologist—to act as an adult "should" and be responsible and protect children, to intervene or tell another teacher and lose the trust of her informants? To casually suggest another teacher might like to walk through the cloakroom? To ignore and thus condone the behavior? Yet Christensen is also aware of the privilege she had been granted, to be "let into" the secret world of boys, usually inaccessible to adults; here was an opportunity for deeper understanding of children's social worlds but also a desire to reciprocate the trust that had been given with loyalty. Christensen asks the boy on the floor if he knows how to stop this if he wants to, and Danny says he does, and the other boys confirm that at that point they will let him go. She walks away; eventually the boys emerge from the cloakroom, apparently the best of friends again, their game over.

This encounter ended up significantly shaping the direction of her research, and Christensen reflects on a number of ways in which her experience problematizes notions of adult and child and ethical research. She notes that the event from the child's perspective did not fit within adult dichotomies of "nice" and "nasty," nor did it align with adult conceptions of children's relationships with one another, and with adults. In the position Christensen found herself, the event shed light on cultural expectations of the responsible and protective adult and vulnerable children, while demonstrating how these adult perspectives are not necessarily shared by children. But of most relevance to my discussion here, the encounter problematized the nature of exchanges between researcher and informants and highlighted a conflict between children's cultural values of peer trust, loyalty and comradeship, and adults' cultural values of adult responsibility and protection.[2] This is where child research becomes politically thorny: the reality that children do not conform to adult expectations of what childhood should be confronts the expectation that the responsible adult will police these instances in which children slip out of what children should be. This adult role is what makes children's secret worlds secret, and what makes these so challenging for the adult researcher to access.

My introduction to this secret world, and the political challenges that came with it, accompanied the relationship shift from participant to friend—a transition that Dominguez (2016) notes already raises ethical questions in research with adults, let alone children. My inclusion in the wider network was gradual and happened with some children before others. One day ten-year-old Pikau was asking me to sit next to her on the mat; a few days later another girl was, and then a socially ostracized boy, and a couple of weeks after that another group of girls were making room for me to sit down. So when one morning I arrive at morning tea and am invited to sit with a group of girls while they eat, I think nothing of it. I am curious about the particular combination of girls, since the group includes Pikau, who did not have strong friendships when I first arrived, and Eponi, who lingered at the periphery of groups, but also Ruby and Tiana, whom I have always observed with the popular girls in the class. After the bell rings for playtime, they invite me to join them. "What are you doing?" I ask. They tell me they are just hanging around and talking and singing. We lounge around the side of a building and sing some of the latest pop songs and then some Māori *waiata* (songs). As the bell rings and we head back to the classroom, I ask Pikau why Tiana is playing with us. "She broke up with her friends," comes the reply.

At lunch, I am invited to join the group again. Thinking it will be more of the same hanging out and singing, I come along. Instead, I am told we are play-ing "dares." This is a familiar game from my own childhood, and I quickly pick up the rules of this version; we all simultaneously throw a "paper-scissors-rock," and if only two of the three hand signals are thrown, then the victors get to "dare" the losers. I am curious about the game and interested to see how the dares compare with those from when I was a child. It becomes apparent that the girls' dares are mostly focused on daring a girl to "ask out" a boy—usually an unappealing boy—and if he says "yes," the girl will have to "go out" with him (be his girlfriend).

I am aware that the adults at the school would not view this as appropriate play. A few weeks prior, Mrs. Randell had given the class a stern lecture about how she didn't "want to be hearing any more of this boy-girl nonsense. You're all far too young for that." Yet I also know that these sorts of themes are an impor-tant part of children's cultures—I remember them from my own childhood—a kind of "revolt of the sexual body" (Foucault 1980, 57) in response to societal sup-pression of sexuality in which the disapproval of adults adds illicit associations to the practices, reinforcing them as symbols of in-group status. However, it is one thing for me to turn a blind eye to things I might see as an outside observer; it is another for me to be a participant in things that would be considered inap-propriate from the perspective of adults. I find I am unsure about where the line is, and whether I can "semi-participate" or whether I need to withdraw from the game completely, and lose my in-group status as a consequence. When I lose the paper-scissors-rock game, I say to the group, "Hang on a second, girls, I need to talk to you about something first."

They gather around, and I say, "You know I'm here from the university to do research with you guys, right?"

"About asthma," says Pikau.

"Yup, that's right. So I have to be a bit careful about what I do because I could get into trouble with the university. So I can't, like, ask boys out or anything."

This explanation is readily accepted by the girls, who decide my dare will be to "twerk." I have no problem with making a fool of myself, and I go ahead and dance for them with exaggerated effect. They laugh uproariously. When it comes my turn to dare, I carefully keep my dares benign: dance around the courts saying, "I am a beautiful ballerina, watch me twirl," and go into the playground and sing the school song. These seem to be acceptable dares and get shouts of approval from the girls who are not on the receiving end, while the girls who have to carry them out blush and squirm and complete the dares in shame. I am curious about their behavior, which contrasts with the attitude I had taken to my own dare. The dares are mildly embarrassing but not hugely so, and most other students aren't even paying attention.

Throughout this process I am experiencing a mixture of feelings: unease about whether it is OK for me to participate in this way, delight that I am being included, and fascination with what function this game is serving and what meaning it has for the participants. I am conflicted by my desire to be accepted, my anthropological interest in the interaction, and my unease with playing a role other than the responsible adult.

This unease is exacerbated as we sit chatting on a picnic table and a teacher on duty comes by and asks us what we are doing.

"Talking," one of the girls answers.

"Well, that's not what you're supposed to be doing at playtime, is it?" replies the teacher. I watch this interaction, baffled. Are they not allowed to talk at playtime?

"But we're not allowed to talk in class, so we have to talk now," explains one of the girls.

"You need to talk while you're playing, then," instructs the teacher. "Go and play tag or run some laps."

I am silent, stiff and bewildered about these strange rules I am not aware of, and wondering what the teacher is thinking of me. We move off, as if to do as the teacher said, but then double back and walk into a new area of the playground to continue our game. I have lost the round of paper-scissors-rock, and it is my turn to be dared.

"You have to go and twerk in the bathroom and you can't stop until I say so," orders Ruby. I am taken aback by this dare—it is clearly calculated to push me much further than the last one I did. I am uncomfortable with going into the bathroom; I am not sure if I am allowed to be there as an adult. I have not had the rules explained to me. Most adults would not find themselves in this situation.

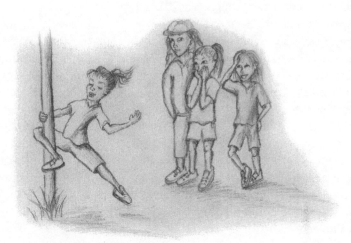

FIGURE 1 Playing dares at Tūrama School.

Ruby laughs at my uncertainty and pushes me into the bathroom. I suddenly realize the importance of shame—and the performance of shame—as central to this game. I did not display a sufficient level of shame the last time I did the twerking dare, and as a result the girls are significantly upping the ante. I quickly perform a half-hearted dance and escape the bathroom, proclaiming my embarrassment. Despite the complaints from Ruby that she "hasn't said stop yet," my performance is met with approval. Although I don't complete the dare, the actions meet their purpose: to shame me and, as such, demonstrate my belonging to the group.

The next child dares Ruby to dance around a pole like a stripper (Figure 1). She does so with a finesse clearly learnt from music videos. My adult self is shocked; my child self wants to try it, too. The other girls show off their pole-dancing moves, and the bell rings.

After school finishes, I drive home uneasy about my level of participation but also fascinated by what I have witnessed. What *was* that? By the time I get home I have a theory; the emphasis on shame and performance suggests I have got myself caught up in a kind of initiation process for a newly forming group.

The next day, after a prize-giving assembly, the deputy principal adds an announcement reminding the children they should be playing a game or doing something active at lunchtime. I realize this is where the duty teacher yesterday was coming from and that I had been inadvertently undermining the school's attempt to regulate the children's free time. Yet knowing this puts me in an awkward position when at lunch I am again invited to play with Pikau, Ruby, and Tiana, and they clearly have no intention of complying with instructions. I go along with them again, but I am nervous of a duty teacher seeing me and thinking I am condoning or encouraging their inappropriate play.

Today Eponi is not with us. I ask the others where she is. "We're not friends with her anymore," came the reply. "She didn't do her dares and she complained, so we kicked her out of the group." This must have occurred earlier, at morning tea. The absence of Eponi tells me that I might be right about my thinking that this dare game is a kind of initiation process. The game starts again immediately after we finish eating, and I make a performance of reluctantly letting them laugh at me twerking again (this time I decline to go into the bathroom) and suggest a few dares of my own when it's my turn: "Do a handstand on the grass." One of the dares is to "flap your arms and say, 'I am a retard.'" "Aw, that's mean," I say, but I don't comment further on the language.

The game seems to run its course, and, having served its purpose of establishing us all as group members, is retired. To my relief, we just hang around a picnic table and sing waiata for the rest of playtime. I am able to Google the words to songs on my phone and am conscious of the social capital I hold as an adult who is allowed to carry a cellphone.

The unease that lingered after the bell rings reflects the disjuncture among the way adults expect children to be, the way children actually are, and expectations about the way adults are supposed to relate to children. I felt uncomfortable being witness to children's games that did not match the adult idea of what is appropriate play, including play that explored themes of shame, power, and sexuality, and uncomfortable that I was observing and participating rather than discouraging or policing. This was the first of many occasions when I had to navigate such political awkwardness. Yet I had learnt more about these girls in two lunchtimes than I had in the preceding weeks of peripheral observation. Although at Tūrama School there was an especially stark difference between how adults wanted children to behave and how children actually are, in any fieldwork with children the adult researcher role has potential to create problems with consequences greater than just discomfort. The times and places at which this issue manifests may usefully highlight adult cultural conceptions of childhood in different contexts, but the challenge is to navigate these moments without giving primacy to these adult conceptions and while maintaining good relationships with both adults and children.

The Transparent Guest

The experience of this event shaped my approach to the remainder of my fieldwork through the discovery that *transparency* about the rules of my role was an effective way of placing boundaries where I needed to. While being "transparent" or "see-through" in a fieldwork context may connote the problematic idea of the invisible researcher, etiologically "transparency" means quite the opposite: to shine light through, to be easily seen—an unmasking of the ethical and social rules guiding the researcher's practice. When faced with the possibility of dares that could put me in a compromised position, simply explaining my position to the girls gave me a legitimate explanation for nonparticipation. While on the first day I was caught by surprise and let myself be pushed into the bathroom, on the second day I was able to explain that I was not allowed in the bathroom and that I might get in trouble with my university and maybe wouldn't be allowed to come to their school anymore. In this, I took on a new role as "transparent guest," openly acknowledging my outsider status and using the norms that the children themselves understood to negotiate my position and justify my actions. With the guest role comes an established set of shared rules that children themselves understand well. Guests, ideally invited, enter and observe in order to learn and follow the rules and cultural practices of the host. But guests may also be exempt from some house rules, or understood as naive about host rules and practices, and so transgressions are more easily forgiven, although if some rules are broken the guest may not be invited back. Guests may also be bound by their own rules brought from home, and in children's culture, "my family say I'm not allowed" is a valid excuse for nonparticipation. As a guest, I could move in and out of different contexts, adapting to the new norms and rules as appropriate. I was sometimes a guest adult, but when invited, I could also be a guest child. Of course, guests are also seen as special, at least initially, but over time and with frequency of visits can become mundane, "like family," and see more "realness" from the hosts.

As a principle, "being open and honest" is generally applied in terms of transparency around research: aims, funding, implications (Price 2016). Here I extend transparency into relationships: as much as possible making the rules that govern my behavior visible so that they are understood and predictable, and in doing so, respecting my participants' competency. I also took this approach with adults in the field. While other authors note struggles with adult gatekeepers and authority figures, few seem to address these directly, as if the researcher's approaches must be kept secret. Shortly after this first event, I attended a staff meeting and took an opportunity to explain my role in the school in more detail, including the explanation that I might sometimes do things that look strange or unusual, because I was trying to get alongside the children as much as possible. I also invited the staff to approach me directly if there were any questions or concerns about what I was doing. After this, my discomfort about playing with the children was much reduced, and sometimes talking through my ethical quandaries with teachers (for example, how I should respond when children begged food off me) seemed to help legitimize my behavior as well. As a model for research with children, the transparent guest role positions ethnographers as actively negotiating and renegotiating complex rules, including those that implicitly and explicitly govern the researcher, in the most visible way possible in order to minimize ambiguities and forestall many of the tensions that can arise from perceived deviancy in practices.

Harmful Implications

Transparent acknowledgement with participants of the rules researchers operate under is also important when considering a second problem arising from an
ambiguous researcher role. Existing categories of adult identity come with known
and predictable sets of rules that are politically important for assisting children
to navigate the adult world. In separating themselves from these categories,
researchers enter uncharted territory not only for themselves, but also for their
participants, who are learning how to interpret and respond to this new kind of
adult. As others have noted, researchers demonstrate their role to child participants through their actions; like others, I recited the mantra "I am not a teacher,
go tell a teacher" until children learned that I would not intervene in their disputes or tell off rule-breakers. Another significant way that I expressed my "different" adult role was by transgressing a simple norm and sitting on the ground
with children, rather than in chairs with adults. In this separated world, my
behavior was not disapproved of—at least not overtly—but it was certainly
noticed. When I sat with the class on the courts to watch an athletics competition, I was asked numerous times if I would like a child to be sent to fetch me a
chair. When I sat on the floor of the school auditorium with the classes waiting
for the bus to arrive to take us on a field trip, teachers and parents all suggested
I might like to sit in a chair. "I like sitting on the floor" became my stock explanation, and before long the children were explaining to adults, "She likes to sit
on the floor." I was seen as odd and unusual, but also there was an understanding that as an anthropologist, it was acceptable for me to do strange things. From
the children's point of view, the simple act of sitting like them seemed to signal
that they could act in their normal ways.

However, because these "differences" are constructed, negotiated, and
learned through interaction in situ, not everyone in the setting—including the
researcher—holds a consistent, complete understanding of the researcher role.
In adopting a role outside of social norms, researchers inevitably will encounter
misreadings, misunderstandings, and tensions from both adults and children.
Discussion of such problems in the literature has done little more than acknowledge these, focusing on how they might cause discomfort for the researcher
who receives funny looks or jokes from adults, or loss of positive relationship,
for example, when researchers have declined or avoided helping adults in the
field (e.g., Mandell 1988). Thorne (1993) worries that by participating—or even
simply declining to intervene—in children's rule-breaking she is undermining
teacher authority and the social order of the classroom.

Less acknowledged is the potential for real harm caused by the ambiguity
of the researcher role to others in the field. Mandell describes an incident in
which she became so lost in the "least adult" role that she neglected to intervene when a child cut open another child's head with a spade. Mandell focuses

on her embarrassment at the scolding she receives from the teacher on duty and how quickly she was forgiven. She does not question whether her presence as an adult meant that the teacher did not step in as soon as she might have had she seen only a group of preschoolers, or if other adults patrolled the area she was in less closely. She also didn't comment on what her prompt pardoning indicated about her privileged position in the day care center, or who ultimately bore responsibility for the injury.

The problem with setting aside the normal rules of known categories of adults is that the limits of this role are not made clear until they are reached in the moments of enactment. While visibly forgoing some of the usual rules of adults, I would still abide by others. From the perspective of the children, this behavior must have seemed quite arbitrary and may have made me difficult to predict. Where this issue became most apparent was when I became privy to talk or behavior that children would routinely keep from adults in order to avoid adult intervention—notably, instances of abuse ("hidings"), suicidal ideation, or self-harm. On the one hand, this is the aim of child research—to get at those hidden practices and develop a child-centered understanding of their world. On the other hand, children keep those worlds hidden for a reason, while I am ethically bound to reveal these incidents. The problem was not deciding whether or not to break confidentiality in each instance, although this was difficult, but in realizing that I might be coming into this information in the first place only because I had set myself up as someone who did not follow normal adult rules. I was in essence misleading children about how they could expect me to respond in other situations.

This problem erupted into my awareness when during an interview with two boys, nine-year-old Whetu cheerfully described how he didn't care when he got hidings from his mother with a pole, with a belt "with the metal bit on top," and with a broom "and the broom broke." Relaxed and chatty, he seemed unaware of the implications of his disclosure for me; when I asked if anyone else knew, he listed a group of friends, "just people that won't tell."

Physical punishment of children has been illegal in New Zealand since 2007 (Crimes [Substituted Section 59] Amendment Act 2007). Most children are well aware of this and also infer that if their parents are reported, they may be jailed and the children removed from their parents' care. As practices of physical force still persist in many homes, this awareness puts many children in the awkward position of protecting their parents even while suffering. The children of Tūrama School are very familiar with CYF, the agency responsible for the protection of young persons under seventeen years old. On one occasion in the classroom I overhead one child correct another on the proper preposition: "you don't go to CYFs, you're with CYFs." This linguistic familiarity reflected the high level of contact CYF had with children at Tūrama School—CYF workers also frequently visited the school as part of interventions with families. CYF is less familiar to children in less challenged circumstances—the agency was never mentioned in interviews with similarly aged middle-class children during my master's research (Spray, Floyd, Littleton, et al. 2018), for example.

The point is that by eight or nine years of age Tūrama School children are well versed in the consequences of letting information slip to adults in the school, and either have themselves been (or are currently) under CYF care or have heard from peers about the consequences of CYF involvement. As well as fears of being "taken away" to live with strangers, children fear getting their parents in trouble, and retribution or shame for betraying their family. As a result, children tended to be circumspect, and although talk of "hidings" was ubiquitous, it was always generalized, or talk about someone else. The school social worker, Lucky, would liaise with families who consented, and reports to CYF were made when necessary to uphold legal obligations.

Unbeknownst to Whetu, I was bound by my university ethics agreement, as well as human responsibility, to act on the information. Despite my obligations I agonized over what felt like a betrayal of this child's trust, of breaking the "children's code." I did not take Whetu's bravado at face value; if his intention was to shock and impress, there were also indications of distress underneath the smiles: "But it's crying," he said, to laughter from his friend Jackson. He cried, but his options constrained, he coped with talk about how little he cared. But, in the moment, with his filter off, he did not make a conscious decision to disclose that information in full knowledge that, in my role as adult, the information would be passed on. I had spent the whole year demonstrating how I was not like other adults; I would tolerate or even laugh at their swearing and dirty jokes; eat their forbidden lollies; shrug off talk of mischief, gangs, and stealing; and turn a blind eye to graffiti or vandalism. Although my participant information sheets said I would break confidentiality for safety concerns, why would a nine-year-old remember that after months of experiencing me in this different kind of adult role? I felt I had misled him, and now if his situation worsened it would be a direct result of my naivete.

If this were an isolated incident, it might be easier to think that Whetu did want me to know and did understand the consequences, or that this was a rare and unfortunate side effect, perhaps even in the child's best interests. Although this was the most serious incident, there were a number of other occasions on which children disclosed information to me that I am confident they would have been more cautious about revealing to another adult. Later in the year a number of girls showed me self-harm marks and then, upon seeing my adult-like response, begged me not to tell a teacher (I told). I also flagged concerns after another disclosure of "hidings" by another boy's father.

In the case of Whetu, I decided that since my lack of transparency had led to the disclosure, I should at least be transparent about what I was going to do about it—even if it cost me rapport with him and probably his friends. I asked to pull him outside of class one day, and while he wound himself around the veranda post and avoided eye contact, I explained that I was concerned about what he had told me and that it sounded like his mum might need some more help, and how would he feel about talking to Lucky about what was going on. Still looking everywhere except at me, Whetu smiled and said Lucky was cool. "Can I go now?" He made a rapid escape, and I figured he'd never speak to me again. I did not learn where the matter went after I gave the details to Whetu's class teacher to be handled privately through school channels. I was surprised, though, when a few weeks later Whetu and his friend Leo (who had until now largely ignored me) came running to meet me before school, dragging me around to visit friends and classrooms, and to play basketball. My popularity with the pair continued for the rest of the year. It appeared I had earned rapport rather than lost it in this instance. There can be an ambivalence in children's relationships to authority; adults offer the potential for options children cannot access on their own, but at the expense of control and carrying the fear of over- or under-response. It seemed that my actions with Whetu had situated me in the "right" kind of adult category. For these boys, caught between craving and fearing adult attention, my interventions may have ended up being more helpful than harmful, although I don't really know, and a positive outcome in this situation does not preclude the potential for harm next time. The problem I am concerned with is the degree to which I found myself in a position of my own making, taking away children's agency and autonomy when they were likely not aware of the consequences of their disclosure. The nature of the issues children at Tūrama School deal with makes this a higher-stakes problem than what might be encountered at a middle-class school, but similar dilemmas could be created in research any place where great discrepancies in power exist between adults and children.

Conclusion

Dilemmas and tensions stemming from generational differences are commonly noted by child researchers, in passing comments or cataloging of challenging experiences. Yet these have not tended to be the subject of analysis to unpack questions about why these tensions emerge, what they tell us about childhood and adulthood, and what role the researcher plays in their creation. Nor is there much discussion of what researchers should do, how conflicting responsibilities may be weighed, and the implications of various responses. How does the way the researcher role is negotiated create new ethical tensions? Whose concept of childhood are researchers using in decision-making, and is this because that concept is the most ethical or simply belongs to the most powerful? When researchers choose to walk away from rule-breaking or taboo play, rather than observe, participate, or police, what impact does this have on their relationships with their child participants and the adults working with those children?

My intention in this chapter was to go beyond acknowledging difficult circumstances in fieldwork by clarifying how and why these difficulties arose, considering the nature of adult-child relationships in this context, how childhood and adulthood are conceptualized, and how children perceive and engage with adult roles. In doing so, my aim is not to solve these issues—I do not think they can be solved—but demonstrate how thinking about generational issues in fieldwork through a relational framework can help researchers better understand the implications of their role and find small strategies—like transparency—to mitigate these difficulties.

Having established the context for this study, and the methodological processes challenging data collection, I now turn to an analysis of children's health coproduction at Tūrama School and surrounding community. The subject of child and adult identities continues in chapter 4, where identities manifest in authority structures and relations of care within the school that shape children's practices of the body in patterned ways. The nuanced understanding of child and adult relations I gleaned from having to work within those relations has therefore also come to have significance for understanding the dynamics of children's health.

4

Coproducing Health
at the School Clinic

In this chapter I begin to answer the main question of this book: How do children participate in the coproduction of their health? As discussed in chapter 1, the anthropology and sociology of childhood literatures have long established that children produce cultural understandings and practices in relation to health and the body (Bluebond-Langner 1978; Christensen 1999; Clark 2003; Mayall 1993, 1996; Prout 1986; Prout and Christensen 1996). This literature has not always captured the processes through which these understandings and practices are guided or constrained by the structures of society, nor the ways in which these structured practices come to shape children's health in patterned ways. In this chapter[1] I build on this literature by elucidating some of the processes through which children's meaning-making and practices articulate with, and are structured by, the institution and state health interventions. I center on the Tūrama School clinic for rheumatic fever prevention and related media campaigns as an entry point for addressing how children engage in interpretive practices in relation to adult-child relations, the body, the school institution, and public health policy, and how these practices, in turn, can shape children's health.

Fundamental to answering the questions of this book is the context of children as peers within an institution marked, as discussed in chapter 3, by distinct power structures separating child and adult roles, rules, and authority. Importantly, schools are also the site at which the state has arguably the most direct relationship with children, since the curriculum and daily activities are to a large degree guided by state policy and interventions targeting "at-risk" children are strategically implemented to maximize efficiency of reach (Burrows and Wright 2007). The story of how children come to creatively appropriate a clinic into their social practices and produce new understandings of illness is therefore also a story of how adult-child relations in the classroom can influence the implementation of state health services, and of how a public health policy can restructure the processes through which children learn how to experience their bodies. These are complex and multifaceted dynamics, and so in this chapter I touch on themes that will be developed over subsequent chapters: the way children's strategies to stabilize their social position may conflict with adult agendas and perceptions of what child well-being means; the way children's activities bring state policies to life in the field and can powerfully impact their effectiveness; and the way that modes of service delivery can restructure children's interpretations of their body.

In this chapter I focus on two main processes through which children's health is coproduced. First, I elaborate Christensen's (1999) analysis of how children collectively construct illness knowledge by demonstrating how state interventions can restructure this embodied process in such a way that children produce novel understandings of "sore throat" and "rheumatic fever." Second, I explore how, structured by the institutional context of the school, children collectively appropriate the clinic into the formulation of social routines that mediate their engagement with health care. I identify three motivations for these routines, which do not necessarily represent conscious or mutually exclusive strategies. First, as navigating peer relations is a salient concern of children (see chapter 7), children can appropriate the clinic into strategies of relationship-building. Second, children's agendas can often conflict with those of adults, creating tension between authority structures and resistance that can result in stressful classroom environments, so that children may use the clinic as a place of respite. Third, by creating social routines of "getting out of class," children may also be creating new ways to legitimize access to health care while maintaining "tough" reputations among peers. Both children's creative conceptions of illness and the social routines they construct around the clinic mediate the ways they access health care from the clinic and, on occasion, their use of pharmaceuticals and other health practices—key ways in which children contribute to the coproduction of their health.

"Who Has a Sore Throat?"

It is the end of summer in my early days of fieldwork, and children entering the classroom after the morning bell are breathless and sticky from an early game on the field before school. Mrs. Randall's classroom is brightly decorated with student artwork, carefully mounted on black cards, labeled with teachers' neat round handwriting, and pinned on the wall or pegged on strings that bisect the airspace above us. As we do every morning, we sit on the mat, a large carpet on an open area of the floor. I sit toward the back so my looming body does not block the view, and children slip snugly on either side of me even though there is lots of room, leaning against me, their bodies damp and hot. As Mrs. Randall takes the roll, Jackson and Aaron are pinching the sides of the boys sitting in front of them. The boys flinch and try not to squeal, keeping their faces trained to the front so as not to draw their teacher's attention.

"Who needs to order a spare lunch?" Mrs. Randall asks, and writes down the names of two children on a paper form. "And who has a sore throat?" More than a third of the hands go up. I glance at Mrs. Randall to see whether this response is normal, but she is already writing down the names.

"Whetu, take this to the office please, darling," Mrs. Randall says, handing him the forms.

A couple of latecomers slip into the classroom: Verity and her younger sister, Karina. Mrs. Randall's eyes widened. "Why are you two late?" she exclaims. Karina looks embarrassed, but Verity shrugs. "Our mother was late," she says. Mrs. Randall looks like she might say something further, but at that moment another latecomer appears at the door. Mrs. Randall appears to reassess the battle and only sighs.

"All right. We are going to work on our sample books now," she says. Several children, including Verity, bounce up and head for their desks. "Did I tell you to go?" Mrs. Randall barks, and they pivot, Verity dragging her feet and looking at the ceiling. Everyone sits down again.

"Now you may go—" and there is a mass break for the desks, overwhelming Mrs. Randall's shouts for them to go *quietly* and *stop running!*

The desks are organized in mixed-gender groups, facing each other to form a table, and I take an empty desk next to Caleb, who has started writing in his sample book using a thick, intoxicating black marker pen. Several times a term, the students complete a piece of work to be sent home to the parents, showcasing their learning, and Mrs. Randall has given me a stack of the sample books to mark for spelling. Jackson, nearby, is swinging on his chair and making electric guitar sounds.

"Be quiet!" Mrs. Randall snaps at the class, and there is a moment of silence before a dull hum resurfaces. Their sample book worksheets for term one are called "My School" and the children have to copy out the school expectations and answer questions about themselves: things they have achieved; how they can demonstrate responsibility; ways they could be fair or not fair; who their role models are. The children at my table hold pencils over their workbooks and chat about their families. "My mum has too many kids," says Cassidee. I tune in and out of their conversation. Her mother is forty-five years old. In the book I am marking, Whetu has supplied an example of when he has been fair: "My sister drew on my face when I was asleep so I drew on her face when she was asleep."

"Jackson, be quiet!" Mrs. Randall shouts, and the electric guitar noises pause, then resume.

At the morning tea break, Cassidee sits by me. She has a large sore on her finger: an inflamed, pus-filled bump. I say, "Ooh, what's that?" because it looks painful. Cassidee shrugs, moves her hand out of view, and continues eating her chips. Her classmates are talking about chili pepper. "I ate some one time and it was so hot!"

"My sister woke me up once, because I was sleeping with my mouth open—"

"—I drank some water but it didn't help—"

"—because I had a blocked nose—"

"—and I was sweating—"

"—and my sister put chili pepper in my mouth and I woke up because it was burning!" We all laugh.

Back in the classroom, we do our spelling and times tables. I do the tests with them, but I don't have to read out my result for Mrs. Randall to record in her big book like everybody else. "Mason—*Jackson*, be quiet!" Mrs. Randall barks; Jackson stops banging his heels on the floor and starts humming instead. "Nine," says Mason.

"What?" says Mrs. Randall.

"Nine," Mason repeats.

"You only got nine out of twenty?"

"Yes," says Mason. His ears are pink.

"How can you only get nine? These are the ten and eleven times-tables. The easiest ones! *Jackson*, be quiet!"

"The sore throat lady is here!" someone calls out, and Mrs. Randall throws up her hands and asks, "Who do you want?" Whaea[2] Allison, the "sore throat lady," reads out the names, and the children disappear out the door. I can see them through the window, running across the courts.

Rheumatic Fever and the Tūrama School Clinic

"Rheumatic fever is a big problem out here," the principal had said to me in our first meeting before I started fieldwork. It was late 2014, and the clinic had been newly installed in a disused classroom, part of the government's 2011 Rheumatic Fever Prevention Programme (RFPP), described in chapter 2, to address rising rates of the disease among low-income Māori and Pasifika children. The clinic's role is to swab children who present with sore throats in order to test for strep throat, the most common form of the GAS infection that can lead to rheumatic fever (Lennon, Peat, Kerdemelidis, et al. 2014). Children diagnosed with strep throat are prescribed a course of antibiotics, usually delivered by parents at home, with a sticker chart that functions both to incentivize children to take the medicine and also to assist families and the clinic staff to track its administration. Occasionally the nurses at school will administer children's antibiotics when there are issues with adherence or when families do not have a refrigerator in which to store the liquid.

Around half the children turned up positive results for strep throat in that initial sweep, the principal told me—a statistic other teachers echoed. By the time I joined Mrs. Randall's class in 2015 the clinic processes had become integrated into the routine of the day. "You should be looking at rheumatic fever," one of the teachers advised, and within a few weeks of fieldwork, I had gained consent from the clinic staff and their manager to observe the clinic. On days when I was based in the classroom, I would follow the children with sore throats to the clinic; on other days I was based in the clinic and would act as runner for Whaea Allison, taking her list to each class and following the stampede of children back. The clinic staff also kindly offered me use of the clinic space to conduct some of my interviews, since the room was empty after school and quieter and more private than regular classrooms.

Not all schools in New Zealand have a sore throat clinic. Most school clinics are located in the Manukau or Northland regions, where rheumatic fever rates are highest in Aotearoa. The Tūrama School clinic is one of sixty-one operating out of schools across Manukau, targeting children deemed demographically at risk—Māori or Pacific children in the lowest deciles of socioeconomic deprivation (Anderson, King, Moss, et al. 2016). The school swabbing program operates in partnership with local providers and, with the consent of parents, approximately 95 percent of Tūrama School children were enrolled in the throat-check program at the time of my research. Whaea Allison, the whānau support worker or "sore throat lady," as the children call her, swabs the children to test for strep throat, while Deb, a registered nurse, attends to positive results: liaising with parents, supplying prescriptions, visiting homes to drop off medicine if the parents cannot get to the pharmacy, providing information and support. In order to maximize swabbing efforts, the clinic has a two-pronged process. Every day, teachers ask the children in the class if they have a sore throat as part of a suite of routine administrative activities, while twice a term, Allison checks the throats of all children in each class with a flashlight and sends those with red or swollen throats to the clinic for a swab. Some of the teachers don't always remember to ask about sore throats every morning, and at times Allison has spoken with teachers to let them know their class came back with a high number of positive results in the class check, and to remind them of the importance of asking for self-identified sore throats. Mrs. Randall, however, is consistent and structured with her routine; she takes her role in the fight against sore throats seriously, and just as well, because sometimes up to half of the children put up their hands to be swabbed.

While the clinical and political implications of rheumatic fever policy are to greater and lesser degrees the subject of policy attention, what is missing from official accounts of rheumatic fever distribution and subsequent health are the experiences, perspectives, and activities of children themselves. Indeed, while the design, implementation, and ongoing evaluations of the RFPP components have involved parents and caregiver perspectives, children fade into the background of these documents (Anderson, King, Moss, et al. 2016; Ministry of Health

2013; Ministry of Health 2015; Vermillion Peirce, Akroyd, and Tafuna 2015): the passive sufferers of disease and recipients of care. As a result, the program reflects parents' understandings, concerns, and barriers to care, but children's experiences and perspectives are largely invisible. For example, evaluations recognize that parents do not typically think of children's sore throats as requiring a visit to a doctor and that standard practice is for parents only to "keep an eye on" their child (Ministry of Health 2013). A large component of the promotional campaign has therefore been to emphasize that sore throats can kill. "It's not cool to take the risk," goes the poster headline. "Get your child's sore throat checked every time." The sad-eyed child sitting in a hospital surgery on the poster is meant to incite parents to take their child's sore throat seriously, but while the Health Promotion Agency consulted with Māori and Pacific health leaders and tested the campaign on the target audience of parents, the agency did not consider how *children* would view these images (personal communication). Other evaluations include the views of adolescents but not younger children, or only test children's health literacy via survey (noting, for example, whether they have heard of rheumatic fever) while soliciting the full experiences of adult whānau members through focus groups (Anderson, King, Moss, et al. 2016; Ministry of Health 2015).

In rendering children's experiences invisible, what policy and evaluation documents do not capture is the way the sore throat clinic inserts itself into the structure of the day, bringing with it specific notions of roles and responsibility for health care and the constant, reinforced reminders to be aware of the throat. Policy does not anticipate the way that children will appropriate the clinic space into social routines of escaping the classroom, nor how public campaigns will contribute to processes of children's health knowledge production and their understanding of risk and risk prevention. Policy does not consider how the daily practices of throat-checking may reshape children's experience of their body by teaching them to be hyper-conscious of the visceralities of the throat (detailed further in chapter 6).

Likewise, apart from a small component of the RFPP that involves referring some families for housing support (primarily insulation), these studies of socioeconomic disadvantage and disease neglect the well-established impact of psychosocial and homeostatic stress on children's immune function (Haggerty 1986; McEwen 1998), including decades-old evidence that stress may increase the likelihood of strep infection (Meyer and Haggerty 1962). Yet a child-centered perspective can immediately identify how not only structural conditions, but children's interpretive practices mediate the experience of stress in the body, whether through the psychosocial stress generated from peer relations (Spray, Floyd, Littleton, et al. 2018; see also chapter 7), the way institutions structure bodily signals of cold or hunger (chapter 6), or the way children's social practices contribute to patterns of nutrition (chapter 5).

All of these dynamics are embodied through a new habitus of children's co-creation—the social structures and bodily dispositions that in turn guide their practice. In this way, an environment structured to disadvantage this group of children becomes physically embodied via the institution, while children's own practices, based on their interpretive understandings of that embodied experience, work toward generating new structures that guide the coproduction of health. A major government health initiative is connected to Mrs. Randall's classroom environment via the activities of children—activities that also contribute to the social structures that shape children's engagement with health care and practices of the body. In the remainder of this chapter I discuss two of the processes through which children help to co-construct this new habitus: children's embodied knowledge production and children's social routines.

Visiting the Clinic

The days are growing crisp and cool, and with the temperature drop comes a settling into the school routine and an uptick of visitors to the clinic. Not all of the children who say they have a sore throat will be fetched from their classroom for swabbing today, though. With around twenty classes, it is not usually possible to get to everyone, and Allison looks over the names with a discerning eye. "They've just had class check this week," she says of one class. "But maybe him—I don't think he was there." She checks the names recorded in an exercise book. "These three I swabbed last week; they were all negative." This leaves Allison with a list to spend the day working through; she usually gets to about twenty students per day, but because I am here today to help with the running around, she may get through more. She hands me her list for Mrs. Randall's class, with eight or so names, and I make the long walk from the junior school, where the clinic is located, to the block of classrooms on the far side of the courts, past the hall, by the fields. I am greeted at the door with a chorus of "Hi Julie"s. "Why are you here?" asks Mason.

"Quiet!" snaps Mrs. Randall. The Education Review Office is inspecting the school next week, and Mrs. Randall has been in a frenzy getting her classroom in order. I read out the names of the children, who take off out the door.

The clinic classroom is set up with three low tables at the back and a shelf of books and a few toys to occupy children who are waiting for their turn to be checked. For some children, this is a space to be free, muck around, and talk unencumbered by the policing of teachers. If they get too rowdy Allison will reprimand them, but her attention is on the child she is working with, and for the most part the waiting children are left alone until they are called for their turn.

I follow the stragglers into the clinic, where Whaea Allison is finishing up with the last group. The sprinters from Mrs. Randall's class are playing on the "spinning" office chair in the corner, but nine-year-old Dandre heads straight for Whaea Allison's desk, calling out "I'm first!" Five or six others pull over chairs in a semicircle alongside Allison's desk, chatting and joking with her as they watch one another undergo examination. Under the mournful gaze of the two boys in the rheumatic fever poster warning of deaths that started from a sore throat, Dandre weighs himself, helped by other children, and calls out the number to Allison to write down. "Do you have a sore throat?" Allison asks, and he nods, opening his mouth wide for her to check with a small flashlight, and watching as she circles "sore throat" and "redness" on his form. He sits upright, beaming as Allison lets him check his own temperature with the electronic thermometer, and holds statue-still while she swabs the back of his throat—a process all children describe as uncomfortable since it "tickles" and can stimulate gag reflexes (Figure 2). "Well done, Dandre," says Allison; she has a friendly rapport with these children, and Dandre basks under her attention. "Can I go back to class now?" he asks, and waves goodbye to his classmates as he slips out the door.

When the rest of the children in Mrs. Randall's class have gone, Allison sighs. Earlier, she and Deb had discussed a current dilemma—a large number of children who self-identify as having a sore throat on almost a weekly basis but rarely test positive for strep. The problem varies by class, and Mrs. Randall's class, along with a couple of the other senior classes, has one of the largest groups of regular clinic visitors. The main issue is the expense; each swab costs about NZ$15, and Allison feels an obligation to manage government resources responsibly. On the other hand, she doesn't want to dissuade children from coming if they genuinely have a sore throat—the risk of rheumatic fever is real. Yet Allison's suspicion is that many of these children were just here to "muck around" and get out of class. "They go straight down the back going "I'm last"—they're not really here to get their throats checked," she grumbles, although this was not the case with most of Mrs. Randall's class today.

This observation is supported by district-wide evidence showing that while swabbing numbers have increased over the period, the proportion of swabs returning a positive result has decreased (Anderson, King, Moss, et al. 2016). It has been noted in the literature that in regular clinics, patients will fall within a normal range from avoidant to over-vigilant, and studies of school clinics indicate the same pattern. The term "worried well" describes the 5–10 percent of patients who seek health care but who are not unwell (Korbin and Zahorik 1985; Lewis, Lewis, Lorimer, et al. 1977). By comparison, over the first seven months of my fieldwork, around the same percentage of swabs for self-identified children—9 percent of 1,434 swabs (range: 2–20 percent)—came back *positive* for streptococcus A (data provided by Manakidz). This does not mean that 90 percent of the time children are well—there are many other causes of sore throat—but these numbers do correlate with Allison's and my own observations of children in the classroom. While I could not calculate the distribution of swabbing across children at Tūrama School because of privacy issues, the raw number

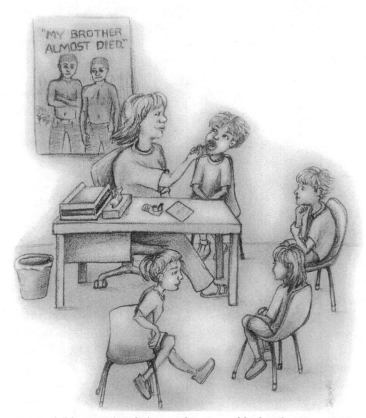

FIGURE 2 Children getting their sore throats swabbed at the Tūrama School clinic.

of swabs the clinic took over the course of my fieldwork—3,159 from both self-identifications and class checks—works out to average seven swabs a year for each child. In other words, children come to the clinic *a lot*.

A few days later, Dandre approaches me and asks why I didn't get him today. Mrs. Randall wrote his name down this morning, he says.

"Because Whaea Allison said you already had a swab come back positive, so she's going to get you some medicine," I answer.

Dandre looks confused. "But I have a sore throat today."

"Mm yes, but did you have a swab a few days ago?"

He looks uncertain. "Yeah, I had a sore throat a few days ago."

"Yeah, so Whaea Deb is going to give your mum some medicine for you."

"But why don't I need to get checked today?"

"Because you already got checked, and you're going to get some medicine soon."

"Julie, come play with us!" Dandre is still frowning as I am pulled away.

Dandre's anxiety on this day is what first prompted me to really wonder about the nature of children's engagement with the clinic. It did not seem as if Dandre just wanted to get out of class, although I could also see what the nurses meant about the children who played and joked and tried to extend their time in the clinic as long as possible. It was not until I began interviewing children later in the year, however, that I could start to interpret how their practices of attending the clinic might be shaping, and be shaped by, their production of illness knowledge.

Learning Sore Throat

Working from an adult model of illness, a basic assumption of the RFPP is that children share an adult understanding of sore throat, and if children have a sore throat, they will know. This is an assumption I initially made myself, and I had some very confused moments in interviews before thinking to ask ten-year-old Anton, "What is a sore throat?"

"Like the fever, you know? Coughs and that, sneezing and that. Cold and that."

After I started asking, I got all sorts of descriptions, some of which represented a traditional or clinical idea of sore throat, but many of which did not. Alzea (age ten) thought the flu and sore throat were the same, associating both conditions with coughing, headache, and blocked or painful swallowing from coughing too much. For Trystan (eleven) a sore throat was "when you're coughing and stuff. And your throat gets hot and that." Navahn (eleven) saw it as an allergy where "you can't eat" and "there's lumps." Meanwhile, children who had connected a painful throat to the label "sore throat" often did not differentiate between sore throats with known causes, such as "talking too much" or "eating scratchy food," from sore throats that could represent a symptom of illness.

The processes through which such understandings of sore throat are produced might be best understood through a conceptual frame that places the experience of the body central to the production of illness knowledge, but also incorporates how the body comes to be interpreted through interactions with others. In her work with Danish schoolchildren, Christensen (1999) provides a theoretical explanation of the processes through which children come to recognize illness. She observed the tendency of children both to bring minor ailments—such as a brief sensation of nausea—to the attention of adults and also to accept or adapt to more serious ailments, like Cassidee's disregard of the sore on her finger that morning tea break. These observations are mirrored in the Tūrama School context, where some children present themselves to teachers and the nurses with "sore throat" on a weekly basis, while other children, identified through a class check to have throats so swollen that the nurses wonder how they can breathe or eat, are seemingly unaware of their condition.

While these two tendencies may seem contradictory, Christensen argues that they demonstrate how these children's understanding of health and illness reflects a process of learning to translate the subjective experience of the "incarnate" body into symptoms and sicknesses according to local cultural classifications and models of body parts and their functioning—the "somatic" body. Christensen draws on the work of Ronald Frankenberg (1980) and Allan Young (1982), who recognize that biological or behavioral signs in the body are interpreted in culturally specific ways and come to be socially recognized as "symptoms" of illness. Christensen adds to this that recognizing unusual signs as illness is not a kind of intrinsic ability that people are born with; rather, children must learn to identify and distinguish signs of illness from other kinds of uncomfortable or unpleasant experiences of the body. The body is normally very changeable, so actors are not necessarily able to recognize an "out of the ordinary" bodily sensation. As children grow up, they come to learn and engage with a complex interpretive and classificatory process of understanding that some bodily sensations of discomfort or pain are accepted as "normal," and others are not.

This learning process involves the conversion of bodily sensations (the incarnate body) into symptoms of illness (the somatic body) through several social processes. When a child brings feelings, injuries, or bodily signs of illness to the attention of an adult, the adult will determine whether the child is "really sick," often using technical equipment such as a thermometer. Once established as sick, adults will administer treatment and separate the child from other children by bringing them to the sick room or keeping them at home. Thus, children link their experience of the incarnate body to its cultural classification, first, through the verification of illness by adult authority and, second, by the symbolic experience of what happens next: staying home, being cared for, drinking or eating certain things, and having medicine. Notably, for Christensen's child participants, being ill means "then I cannot do, what I usually do" (1999, 187), which could be experienced as annoying, but also signifies their illness as a special event. Finally, Christensen observes children engaging with peers in a "collective bricolage of the body" (1999, 210), drawing on social experiences and knowledge of the body to link bodily experiences to the "somatic" body. Such a process can be observed in the Tūrama School children's earlier conversation about the effects of chili pepper on the body. Thus, peer groups make significant contributions toward children's understandings of illness, both as sources of information about bodily experiences and as collaborators in the project of connecting those experiences to cultural models or classification systems.

I suggest that the Tūrama School clinic restructures these processes of linking subjective experiences of discomfort to the diagnosis of illness, resulting in the production of new understandings of illness, in such a way that children are more likely to present to the clinic to be swabbed. This restructuring occurs because the prevention program is primarily based on a subjective symptom—sore throat—and relies on children identifying when they have a sore throat, either by telling their teacher and presenting at the clinic, or by telling a parent so that they may be taken to the doctor to be swabbed for strep throat. This process presupposes that children have acquired an adult conception of the link between the incarnate experience of a painful throat and the somatic understanding of *some forms* of this experience as a symptom labeled "sore throat."

In the school, however, children's somatic understanding of sore throat does not always match the adult biomedical model. Ten-year-old Ngawaina, for example, creates her own terminology to differentiate between her experience of sore throat symptoms and the clinically diagnosed condition that requires treatment:

NGAWAINA: I don't think my throat was . . . *sore* sore.

JULIE: It wasn't sore sore.

NGAWAINA: I don't think so.

JULIE: What's the difference between sore sore and not sore sore?

NGAWAINA: Sore sore is like . . . you really need medicine? And not really sore is when . . . you just need a good night rest?

Compounding the variable understandings of sore throat is a lack of clarity about the difference between sore throat—the symptom—and strep throat as one specific cause of sore throat. Media campaigns focus on sore throat, with little mention of strep throat, while nurses speak of children being "positive," usually without specifying for what. For many children like Ngawaina, sore throat and strep throat become conflated, and sore throat comes to be understood in somatic terms as its own condition, diagnosed by the clinic staff or the lab. As a result, ten-year-old Mila comes to the clinic not because she *feels* a painful throat, but "so the nurse can check if I have a sore throat."

In this context children's "illness" is also being verified by adults in a very explicit and formal way, an institutionalization of the everyday social process in which adults validate children's illness claims, helping them to link the body incarnate to the somatic body. As in Christensen's observations of Danish adults and children, the Tūrama School sore throat checks involve adult devices that demonstrate adult competencies and signify illness. Allison will take the children's temperature, weigh them, look in their mouth with a flashlight, feel their neck glands, and swab their throats. Children pay close attention to the results of these assessments, and in particular the sheet of paper where they are recorded. "And every time I come here, she puts me down as a redness and swollen," Amberlee (age ten) tells me. "Because I watch her, and when she does that it actually kind of freaks me out." Importantly, Allison circles "sore throat" on the form to record children's self-reported symptoms, but for children watching, this action confirms their "sore throat" is real. Children therefore don't need the lab results; the assessment, swabbing, and recording process is in itself the verification that confirms children's bodily sensations—whatever they may be—as sore throat. Hence, "sore throat" becomes not only a subjective experience, but a condition that is externally diagnosed.

To further complicate things, sometimes children don't experience a painful throat but are identified in a class check and swabbed. In such instances, sore throat becomes something that *you might not know you have.* This experience was very powerful for Mila, who had been "given the medicine" (diagnosed with strep throat) multiple times but never experienced a sore throat. "But sometimes I do have sore throats but I don't actually feel it?" she tells me. "So, I'll just think that I've got nothing to worry about?" Because Mila is unable to link her diagnoses with any perceptible symptoms, she presents at the clinic regularly—twelve times this year, she estimated in November—so that Allison can check whether or not she has a sore throat.

Thus, the connections children make between subjective sensations of the body incarnate and the illnesses of the somatic body are reconfigured by the school clinic; any symptoms, even an absence of symptoms, can be verified by medical authorities as sore throat. The incarnate experience of sore throat becomes anything ranging from sneezes to lack of feeling, while the somatic category of sore throat shifts from a symptom to a diagnosis. Unlike the interactions that Christensen observed, Tūrama School children are not simply learning to classify their bodily experiences according to adult concepts of illness but are also creating their own concepts and classifications—sore throat the symptom, and *sore* sore throat the illness—to explain the inconsistencies between their experience and their diagnosis. This creative coproduction of illness concepts continues in the construction of rheumatic fever.

Children's Knowledge of Rheumatic Fever

Two shirtless, solemn boys gaze out from a large poster behind Allison's desk. With a long scar down one of the boys' chest clearly visible, they oversee the children getting their throats swabbed with the message "My brother almost died . . . it all started with a sore throat" and the slogan I had come to hear so often: sore throat leads to rheumatic fever, leads to heart damage. Inside or outside of the clinic, I heard children repeat the messages from the poster and from the related television campaigns.

"Yeah, that ad," said ten-year-old Te Kapua, reciting, "My brother almost died. It started with a sore throat."

Mila tells me how she always likes watching TV, and she likes watching ads, and how "that ad always comes up." In her narrative, though, she adds detail not depicted in the advertisement: a sore throat clinic, a clinic lady, and some medicine that the boy's mother always gave him.

"Well, that little boy? Had a sore throat, and told his mum, and the clinic lady, but the clinic lady had nothing to do, so she just gave him medicine. And his mum always gave the medicine to him. And then . . . suddenly, he started having a sore throat. And like, he couldn't breathe properly? So he got rushed to hospital, and they had to cut him open. And, and cure what—and cure what happened to his throat. 'Cause he had heart damage."

This media campaign (Figure 3) was designed by New Zealand's Health Promotion Agency and includes posters that appear across bus shelters and buildings in targeted areas and a television campaign that has aired since 2014. The campaign was intended to target parents (particularly Māori and Pasifika parents) but also captured the attention of children who identified with the jokey, rugby-playing boys in the video. From what I could tell based on interviews and observation, this campaign formed the primary source of children's rheumatic fever knowledge; little additional information was formally provided to children, although Allison would competently answer children's questions. When the clinic first opened, shortly before I began fieldwork, the clinic staff gave a talk in assembly, but this was not repeated in the time that I was there, and few children ever mentioned anything other than the media campaign as a source of their knowledge. An information packet went home to parents with the consent forms, but this was not written at most children's reading level. The nurse, Deb, gave me a long list of points that she covered with parents when advising of a positive diagnosis and delivering medicine, including storage, adherence, dosage, side effects, reactions, and information for the doctor. When I asked what information Deb gave to the children, the things she listed were reminders—to remind mum and dad to give them the medicine, to bring back their sticker chart—and discussion of their experience of treatment, rather than information.

As a result, children's detailed and developed conceptualization of rheumatic fever was constructed using the media campaign as scaffolding. Across the main elements—the sequence of three conditions, the link to death, the primacy of sore throat—children have (to paraphrase both Corsaro [1992] and Geertz [1973]) spun their webs of meaning, using their own experience and what they observed of those around them, and filling in the gaps that adults left blank with knowledge of the children's own production. Thus, children's conception of rheumatic fever was consistently unified around a model of its etiology—the most salient aspect. This model was expressed in three stages (or four, with the fourth stage being death), and some children explicitly referred to numbered stages.

During an interview in the clinic classroom after school, three ten- and eleven-year-old girls tell me what they know of rheumatic fever. In a collective bricolage reminiscent of Christensen's description of three Danish children compiling their knowledge of the body's organs (1999, 211–212), they link their experiences and observations of "what happens" and "what you do" to the model of

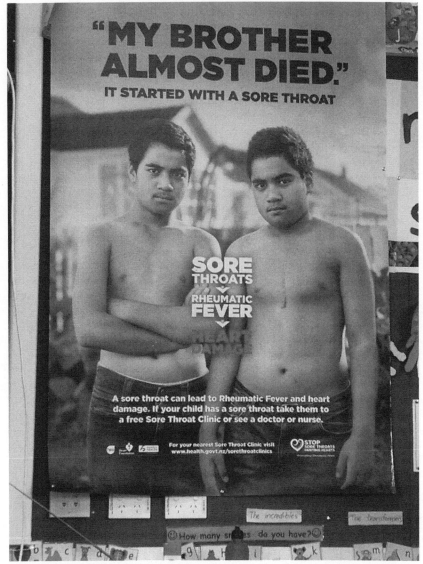

FIGURE 3 Campaign poster for rheumatic fever in the classroom clinic. Poster produced by the Health Promotion Agency of New Zealand. Photograph taken by the author.

illness presented on the poster. Ruby responds first: "Rheumatic fever, 'cause my cousin had it, and he only made it to the second one, and he almost made it to the heart thing, but they . . ." she mumbles, perhaps unclear about what "they" did to prevent heart damage.

"What do you mean, he only made it to the second one?" I ask.

Ruby explains, "'cause like there's three, aye, and you start from sore throat, then you get rheumatic fever, but he never got the things down there." She points to the poster behind her. "Oh, he never got the heart disease," I say, reading the poster.

As Ngapaea and Alexandra, who have been distracted, tune back into the conversation, I ask again:

"What do you know about rheumatic fever?"

Ruby begins, "It starts from a sore throat—" She is interrupted by Ngapaea.

"—Oh, it starts from a sore throat, then it goes to heart damage—"

"—No, it goes to rheumatic fever."

At this point Alexandra jumps in. "It starts with sore throat then rheumatic fever—

"—and then heart damage—" all three girls chime.

"—and then dead," Alexandra finishes.

This way of describing rheumatic fever was ubiquitous among these children. Stage one was the sore throat, which, as described earlier, was represented by a plurality of meanings. Children had a clear idea that if their sore throat was not checked, it could get worse and progress to stage two, rheumatic fever. For most children, stage three, heart damage, was linked to death. As the girls explained:

Ngapaea: "And the reason we have to have sore throat lady here is, she have to give 'em medicine to make—you might have heart damage. We get heart damage, we're gonna have to end up in hospital, and we have to—"

Ruby: "—No, 'cause we can—if—if we too late we can pass away—"

Alexandra: "—And if we get heart damage we'll die."

Rheumatic fever was therefore conceptualized primarily in terms of its relationship to sore throat and heart damage, and in its perceived proximity to death, a linear series that would inevitably progress through the stages if no intervention was to occur. As noted earlier, few children included strep throat in their model, reflecting the absence of strep throat in the media campaigns. Consequently, it seems that many children, after receiving antibiotics, may have inferred that they were now at "stage two" of this model and believed they had rheumatic fever. Several children told me about their past history of "rheumatic fever," but described the experience of having their throat swabbed by Allison or a doctor and taking antibiotics for ten days. "Heart damage, I just had that before. For just like two weeks," Anton tells me. Some of these children would tell me the *doctor* told their mother they had rheumatic fever, so it is unclear whether the communication issue was between doctor and parent, or whether children reinterpreted the information from their parent and attributed their understanding to medical authority.

Yet because children would share their "diagnosis" with their peers, the effect of this was to increase perceptions of the risk of sore throat progressing to rheumatic fever. "Jackson's got rheumatic fever!" an eleven-year-old girl hissed across the classroom when Jackson was called to the clinic to receive his antibiotics. Children would also commonly attribute the illness or deaths of family members to rheumatic fever. Contrary, however, to how rheumatic fever is represented in the media campaign, child death from acute rheumatic fever is extremely rare, although it is possible that some adult deaths may have represented early mortality from the effects of chronic rheumatic heart disease (CRHD). But in many cases, it later transpired that the cause of death had been another illness such as pneumonia. Although actual incidences of rheumatic fever remain relatively rare, and most children are probably not even susceptible, as a collective these rheumatic fever narratives created a sense of the disease as much more commonplace, inevitable, and deadly than the epidemiological data would suggest. By contrast, the one child I knew of in the senior school who actually did have heart valve damage from a prior bout of rheumatic fever hid his condition from his peers. Nine-year-old Victor would tell his class he was in trouble with the principal when he was called to the office to meet the district health nurse who visited Tūrama School to administer his monthly prophylactic penicillin injections.

While children match their experiences and those of their peers to the model presented in the campaign, the process of connecting the incarnate and somatic bodies was also restructured by the spatial marking of illness. Similar to the children of Christensen's study, the Tūrama School children associated the experience of being sick with staying home and taking medicine. Although the nurse told me she would try to explain to parents that children needed to stay home from school only if they felt too unwell to go, several children told me they stayed at home for the entire ten-day duration of the antibiotics course, despite a lack of symptoms. Ten-year-old Cassidee told me when the "doctors" told her mum she had rheumatic fever they said "that I had to stay home for like, two weeks. That was boring." Staying at home had the effect of symbolically marking their experience as illness, and children who stayed at home, like Cassidee, were also more likely to be those who interpreted their illness as "rheumatic fever."

In contrast to the children's models of sore throat, their models of rheumatic fever had less emphasis on symptoms, exactly what the condition is, or how it might be experienced. That the most salient incarnate experience of "rheumatic fever" for Cassidee was boredom makes sense given that any strep throat symptoms probably subsided within a day or two of receiving antibiotics. However, for nine-year-old Marielle, who had given me detailed descriptions of the rheumatic fever campaign, it appears the fear of her diagnosis may have formed her incarnate experience of what she understood to be "rheumatic fever." Even in my interview with her, she gasps between words, unconsciously re-enacting the embodied memory of the illness she associates with breathlessness. "I thought I was gonna die because it was my first time," she tells me. "Rheumatic fever is how . . . um, you can't breathe properly? Well, you can't—well, you can breathe but you can't breathe properly, and um, you get heart damage sometimes, if you're—if you got that very—if you got rheumatic fever too long? And it can be caused by um, sore throats."

Marielle described the breathlessness as starting after she went to the doctor:

". . . like after. And then I was like, thinking . . . what just happened? . . . Then I was thinking, like, I was gonna be that boy [in the campaign]? Like you know, huh, I was like . . ." Her voice shakes, "Ahhhh, I've gotta take my pills!"

The nurse later confirmed to me that strep throat is not associated with breathing difficulties, and Marielle's breathlessness was most likely anxious hyperventilation, perhaps triggered by the thought that she, too, would be like the boy on the poster who almost died. Thus while children construct a somatic understanding of rheumatic fever around a model of its etiology, linking campaign information to their social observations and experiences, they also produce a "rheumatic fever" incarnate, primarily experienced as emotions such as boredom and anxiety, and symbolically marked by staying home and taking medicine.

These processes of illness knowledge production therefore shape children's health practices in several ways. Because of the fear she associates with rheumatic fever, Marielle engages with the clinic more often, and she also becomes vigilant about taking her medicine. Although (with a possible exception being children coping with chronic illness) children's self-administration of pharmaceuticals is often viewed as inappropriate (Mayall 1993; Christensen 1999), other children besides Marielle also engaged in a variety of semi-independent interpretive practices around pharmaceuticals that contribute to the coproduction of their health. For example, medicine can represent a marker of age status for the children of Tūrama School; because the school nurses administer antibiotics in either liquid or tablet form, children have come to create a shared social understanding that liquid medicine is for young children, and pills are for older children. This may be why Victor, rather than asking for liquid medicine, spat his pills into the rubbish bin when he struggled to swallow them.

In turn, the self-administration of medicine reflects adult status—something some children may aspire to or be encouraged toward. Nine-year-old Hinemaia, who earns praise from her teacher for her maturity and responsibility, describes helping herself to her brother's antibiotics from the kitchen when she feels a "fever." The natural extension of enacting that maturity, for Hinemaia, may be taking care of herself pharmaceutically. Likewise, the motherly nine-year-old Teuila, who is Tongan, describes how she diligently takes her antibiotics only every second day so that her younger siblings might have the other half, perhaps enacting an elder sister's care and responsibility.

Children's conceptions of illness can also inform their pharmaceutical practices. Nine-year-old Dandre and his sister Jordyn are regular visitors to the sore

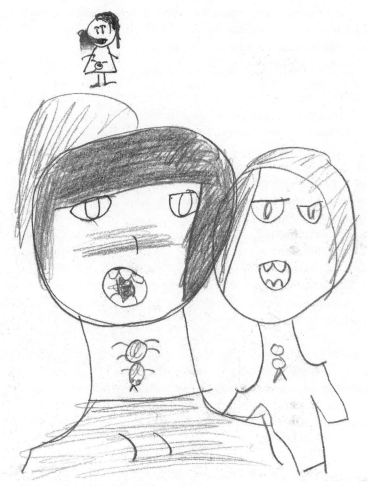

FIGURE 4 "The Sore Throat Bug" by Jordyn, age nine.

throat clinic, where, they explain in an interview with me, "Whaea Allison can check" to see if they have the "sore throat bug." Across the table littered with empty juice boxes, cookie wrappers, paper, and pencils, Jordyn draws this "bug" for me, an insect-like creature inhabiting her throat (Figure 4). When I ask Dandre if he ever comes to the clinic when he doesn't have a sore throat, he tells me "sometimes when . . . oh, only one time, so they could check if my throat was sore."

"What?"

"See if my throat was sore," Dandre repeats.

"You came here to see if your throat was sore? But you didn't have a sore throat," I clarify.

"Yeah," says Dandre.

After Dandre and Jordyn tell me about how medicine kills the "sore bug," I ask what they think could happen with the bug if they don't take the medicine.

"You will die," Dandre announces bluntly.

"Oh!" I exclaim, surprised.

"And you get that—"

"—And you get a surgery—"

"—I wouldn't even like it," they clamor over each other.

I wonder if they come to the clinic because they're worried they might die, and both agree.

"I thought I was going to die when I didn't even take it," says Jordyn.

"You thought you were going to die when you didn't take it . . . ?"

"Yeah," Jordyn explains, "because I forgot to take my medicine, and I thought I was about to die. So I took it."

I clarify; had she just forgotten that day?

"Yeah, so, so I went to go take it again and again," Jordyn explained. "And then I put my sticker on, and I didn't even think about it again."

Dandre and Jordyn's shared conception of the bug in their throat is the product of nurses referring to bacteria as "bugs" and a media campaign that links the bug with death.

However, this conception is a powerful driver of their health practices. Dandre, afraid of the bug that will kill you, goes to the clinic so Whaea Allison can check whether he has a sore throat. Jordyn, panicking that she might die, takes her antibiotics "again and again," before she puts the sticker on her chart to confirm the medicine has been taken, and she can relax once more. Both of these children are therefore active participants in the coproduction of their health, but their creative interpretations are also structured by the socioeconomic conditions that render them vulnerable to rheumatic fever, a health campaign that supplies them with information about the disease, and a health intervention that medicates children rather than changing their conditions.

Getting out of Class

The high numbers of children attending the Tūrama School clinic can therefore be partly attributed to the restructuring of children's knowledge production, through which children collectively generate new understandings of illness and the body to guide their practices. The high numbers can also be attributed to the fear and anxiety generated by a media campaign that features children and talks about them dying. However, Christensen (1999) also describes how moments of illness forefront the very social notions of privacy, intimacy, weakness, and vulnerability associated with feeling unwell. Consequently, illness events accentuate children's social relations—status, hierarchies, relationships—enacted, for example, in whom children notify of an illness event (in Christensen's case, siblings) and who stays by the sick child while he or she receives help (close friends). Illness and health care are therefore closely intertwined with children's peer cultures, in the production not only of knowledge but also of relationships.

The situating of the clinic within the school further amplifies the social nature of health care in this context, and this may also help to explain children's use of the clinic. When I asked about children's reasons for visiting the clinic, most children said that they went to the clinic only to get their throats checked. Several children also complained that teachers sometimes did not believe their sore throat was real and prevented them from visiting the clinic. However, as the nurses suspected, some children did suggest that they or other children went to the clinic to get out of class. This use of the clinic seemed to be connected to Allison's practice of bringing children to the clinic as a class group, rather than individually, which transformed clinic visits into a social event. Amara, a shy nine-year-old who floated at the edge of peer groups, giggled with me that she "sometimes" wants to get out of class; for her, following the more socially successful children to the clinic might have meant an opportunity to strengthen her relationships. Sometimes, "my friends say put your hand up so you can come too," Cassidee told me, but on days when she was the only girl who put up her hand, she would visit the clinic by herself at lunchtime for a swab, rather than go with the boys.

The clinic, therefore, could be appropriated by children into the construction of their social relations. However, clinic visits could also offer a moment of respite from the stresses of the classroom environment. A tension between Mrs. Randall's demands for order and quiet as she tried to accomplish the goals of the state, and the subversive resistance of Jackson, Verity, and other children, created a climate of almost constant conflict that appeared to wear on the children as much as it did me. It perhaps is not surprising, therefore, that large groups of children attended the clinic particularly from Mrs. Randall's class (especially since she asked conscientiously every day about sore throats), as well as that of another teacher with a distinctly authoritarian style.

However, talk of getting out of class could perhaps sometimes function as a discourse for children, particularly those with "tough" reputations, to *justify* going to the clinic to peers. This is where children's illness knowledge production becomes linked to their social routines; it is not *only* that children present to the clinic because they are scared they may have a deadly sore throat, or that children *only* come for the peace and social time. It may also be that children are a little scared of rheumatic fever, but the idea that they visit the clinic to get out of class makes that fear more manageable and makes accessing the maternal care of Whaea Allison more socially acceptable.

Glimpses of these complex dynamics arise in my conversation with eleven-year-olds Trystan and Navahn in their classroom after school one day. The pair, who are best friends and "cousins," because their mothers are cousins, have just inhaled my box of cookies, and Navahn is drawing gang signs with the colored pens and paper I laid out for them to use.

We begin by brainstorming the kinds of illnesses they know about, which in their case is extensive.

"My nan had cancer," says Trystan. "That's how she died."

"My nephew had a asthma attack," says Navahn.

"And I had rheumatic fever," says Trystan.

"And my mum had a epilepsy," says Navahn.

They know about pneumonia because Trystan's auntie just died of it, the class had found out yesterday. She died, Trystan tells me, because she never went to the hospital, because she always drank, and because she didn't take her meds.

"Oh. That must have been really hard to watch. Did you know her well?" I ask.

"She was like my mum," he says. Trystan does not live with his parents.

Rheumatic fever, they know about from the poster in the clinic. "It says my brother had—"

"—rheumatic fever—"

"—ah, rheumatic—oh, and it says, it all started from a sore throat," Navahn finishes.

"You guys have like, memorized that poster," I comment.

Navahn adds, "And one's got a big as, um—my cousin, his name's Lazarus, he's got a big as stitch scar thing there? And that's what he's got on the poster."

The boys estimated they went to clinic about twice a week, the most recent time being that morning. "So how come you're going so often?" I ask.

"To get out of class," Trystan says, and Navahn agrees, adding that too much running around makes them cough.

But they tell me, in great detail, about how they must finish all their antibiotics, which are called amoxicillin, for ten days, because there's twenty pills, so that they won't get rheumatic fever, because last time Trystan didn't take all his meds, he was hospitalized, he says for rheumatic fever. And maybe after today Trystan will be taking the medicine again, if his swab from this morning is positive. "My nephew went positive twelve times this year," Navahn says.

"Has that scared you a bit?" I ask them nonchalantly.

"Yeah."

"Yeah."

"I might get it again," says Trystan.

"Yeah, I'm scared of getting rheumatic fever," says Navahn.

"Are you really?" I ask, a little surprised at their serious tone.

"Yeah. I don't want to go to hospital. I don't want to die," says Navahn. Then he continues, "I'd rather kill myself. Nah, jokes, jokes!" He laughs, grabs my recorder, and apologizes loudly to the speaker, melodrama and mockery steering him away from the edge of vulnerability he has just found himself too far out on.

"Stink-arse," says Trystan.

It is possible that Trystan and Navahn feign a fear of death to cover a well-honed practice of escaping the classroom. But for these boys who live in a world of gangsters and toughness, skipping class may also represent a public excuse to mask a vulnerability that does not fit their staunch social persona. Their expressions in this interview, one moment reflecting on the loss of a parent figure and fear of an illness that seems to saturate their world, the next calling each other names, suggests in themselves an ambivalence about why they are doing what they are doing. If death is an underlying fear turned into a joke, then creating a cultural routine of skipping class also entrenches a socially—and emotionally—acceptable pathway to seeking care.

Conclusion

By December 2016, rheumatic fever rates in Manukau had dropped by a third—a modest success, but not close to the RFPP aim of a two-thirds reduction. The living conditions of families had seen little change, and the problem of child poverty had grown enough to be a primary policy issue in the 2017 elections (Patterson 2017). Meanwhile, Tūrama School children continue to appropriate the clinic processes into their social worlds while, at the same time, the clinic restructures their school day, their knowledge production, and the way they experience their bodies.

This is what is missing from state policy: a view of the embodied, socially embedded practices of children who are collectively carving out a world and their place in it from whatever they encounter. Socialization through the child's eyes, as Allison James (2013) writes, sees children as active players in the process of reproducing culture. Child policy interventions, brought to life in context, are transformed through their social enactment, in interactions between children and the adults who work to care for them. While children's lives can be structured by adult interventions, children also resist, appropriate, or transform those points of contact with the state through tactical and productive practices that make sense in this umwelt, where classrooms are loud, teachers unpredictable, and death appears close.

This is a view instead of a clinic embedded in social relations and power dynamics: between peers, between adults and children, between those in authority and those who are not. In an institution where authority structures mean children have little power over where they go and whom they are with, the clinic may offer a legitimized opportunity for escaping the noise and stress of the classroom. The unusual clinical procedure of examining children in groups also turns health care into a social event, whether children appropriate the clinic as a relationship-building opportunity, or establish social routines of "getting out of class" to make accessing care more comfortable or socially acceptable. These social routines then become a new structure guiding children's engagement with health care.

Generational relations also underpin children's understandings of health and illness, which are constructed in family and school settings where adults validate children's sickness, sometimes using technology such as thermometers, and keep children home in bed or make them go to school (Christensen 1999). When Whaea Allison records children's self-identified sore throat on the form, she verifies children's bodily experiences as symptoms of illness, meaning that sneezing can become sore throat, and sore throat can become something you do not know you have. These processes shape children's patterns of accessing health care in ways that were not predicted by a health policy that does not consider children as significant social actors.

This is Corsaro's (1992) interpretive reproduction, as described in chapter 1: children spinning collective webs of meaning over adult structures and across domains of life. But it is also a generation of culture and practices that are contingent on and constrained by institutional structures and material resources; by the specific social position of children more generally; by childhoods lived in socioeconomic contexts more particularly; and by the physical reality of bodies that are small, cold, sick, growing, hot, hungry, tired, disciplined, emotional. Children play an important and powerful role in their health through the way they respond to these circumstances, whether that be constructing polysemic notions of sore throat as simultaneously symptom and diagnosis, taking their antibiotics "again and again" to make up for a missed day, or generating increased perceptions of rheumatic fever risk through their collective knowledge production and social talk. The processes of coproduction here are therefore the processes that occur between the state and the individual, between structure and agency, between adults and children, and between culture and the body.

5

Responsibilizing Care

In early 2015, just as I was starting fieldwork at Tūrama School, the New Zealand Parliament was debating two members' bills put forward to amend the 1989 Education Act and expand the social services delivered through schools. The first, known as the "Feed the Kids" bill, provided for government-funded breakfasts and lunches in decile 1–2 schools and was defeated 61–59 at its first reading. Debate on the second, the "Food in Schools" bill, which emphasized teaching lifelong nutritional skills, ended in a tied vote, but because a majority is needed, the legislation failed.

The week before the vote on this legislation, I sit on the concrete steps outside a classroom eating my own lunch (Figure 5). As teachers did not eat with their students, I am the only adult among all of the senior children, who must sit outside this particular block of classrooms for the first ten minutes of the lunch break, known as "lunch-eating time." This is a somewhat optimistic epithet, as very few of the children are eating anything more than a packet of chips, if that. "Where's your lunch, Caleb?" I ask the nine-year-old sitting nearby. He shrugs, and gives me the standard response, "I'm not hungry." He accepts a handful of cheese-flavored puffs from Teuila, who sits next to me. This packet of chips is Teuila's complete lunch and she devours them, tipping the crumbs into her mouth and licking her fingers. A staple food for the children at Tūrama school, packets of chips imported from Asia can be bought from the store around the corner for a dollar each, making them significantly cheaper than those produced in New Zealand and, as they come in a bigger packet, an option that can be more liberally shared.

"Julie, what's that?" Teuila asks, looking at my lunch, and I tell her it's a wrap and the filling is chicken and spinach. I had made it myself that morning. "Can I have a piece?" she asks.

"A piece?"

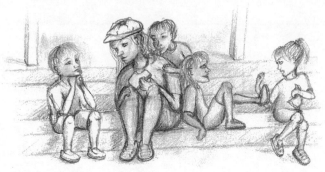

FIGURE 5 Eating lunch at Tūrama School.

"Of that." She points to the spinach.

"You want a leaf of spinach?"

"Yeah." I let her pick one out. How could I not?

I continued eating, enjoying the sunshine and letting my mind drift away from the conversation. As I finished up my wrap, Teuila interrupted my day-dream to ask if she could have the end. Why not, I thought, and handed it over. I didn't need it, and how do you say no to a hungry child, anyway?

"Can I have the end tomorrow, too?"

"Uh . . ." I am beginning to see why the teachers don't eat with the children.

"Or maybe you could bring me one?" Teuila tilts her head to the side and gives me a dimpled smile, but I can see in her eyes that she knows what she is asking for is a little shameful.

"Eh, don't scab,[1] Teuila!" Another child admonishes, buying me time to decide how reply. Teuila scowls in response, but with some embarrassment.

"Hm, I don't know. If I brought another lunch for you, then wouldn't I have to bring everyone lunch? I can't afford that!"

This prompts an argument about how many lunches I should bring.

"Yes, bring all of us lunch!" someone shouts. Other children posit that I should not have to bring any extra lunches.

"You could just bring one extra lunch and give it to one child each day," suggests Caleb. "This morning my dad said tomorrow there would be no lunch. He said we've run out of bread. Will you be here tomorrow, Julie?" he asks hopefully.

This encounter where my lunch was scrutinized, fought over, and shared, was one of many throughout my fieldwork at Tūrama School. While I generally shared when asked, I did manage to solve the dilemma to a certain extent by bringing the most unappealing lunch I could; I discovered that while I liked peanut butter sandwiches on whole-grain bread, the children did not, and my lunch tended to be left alone.[2]

While I was sharing my lunch with "scabbers," Prime Minister John Key, after an informal phone survey of three schools, argued that the number of children coming to school without lunch is relatively low (Young 2015), and for those who are, Minister of Social Development Paula Bennett invoked "parental responsibility" to defeat the proposed legislation that would have supplied all of the children at Tūrama School with a free lunch (Burrow 2015). The members of parliament who voted against the legislation were strongly criticized by the opposition for being "out of touch" and denying the extent of poverty in Aotearoa.

Meanwhile, the perceptions of children themselves were conspicuously absent from these debates. This invisibilization of children's perspectives is routine in child policy, reflecting common assumptions about children as passive recipients of care and provisioning, rather than as social actors who play a role in their own health. Yet, the anthropology and sociology of childhood have repeatedly demonstrated the capacity of children to employ agency in the negotiation of their health (Bluebond-Langner 1978; Clark 2003; Mayall 1993, 1996; Prout 1986), dismantling the notion that adults give care, and children accept it (Hunleth 2017). Studies of children and care have tended to focus on how children exercise agency in their self-care and in *giving* care (Christensen 1999; Hunleth 2017), but less on the conditions under which children do or do not accept care. Yet, as I will argue, the meanings and practices children construct can mediate the effect of care on their health, so it is important to consider the way that children will interpret state and institutional services.

As apparent in the school lunches debate, children's health care in Aotearoa is configured around notions of responsibility that shape the particular ways that the state, institutions, parents, and children are implicated in the delivery of care and provisioning. However, ideas about responsibility for care—who initiates and accounts for what and how care is provided—shift with the positioning of social actors and the state. I have noted the perspectives of teachers of their responsibilities for care of children within the school system in chapter 2; in this chapter I contrast the views advocated by the state, often reflected in public discourse, with the views of children themselves. While these perspectives may overlap or, at times, find congruence, they are not the same, and the differences between how the state sees responsibility for children's care and how this is understood by children themselves can help to explain how and why children engage with different forms of care at school.

Adopting a neoliberal ideology, successive New Zealand governments have discursively allocated responsibility for children's care to parents, while dispelling any state responsibility for the inequitable conditions underlying poverty and ill health. As a result, state services are designed to "support" and "educate" parents to discharge their responsibilities, while gaps are often patched, with varying degrees of adequacy, by community and corporate organizations. Meanwhile, care in childhood is fundamentally embedded in intergenerational processes, and care relations are a key mode through which social positions are enacted and relationships nurtured. If the state conceptualizes care in terms of neoliberal parental responsibility, children see responsibility for care as the enactment of intergenerational and affective relations (Christensen 1999; Hunleth 2017). From the perspective of Tūrama School children, *adults*, whether in families, schools, or communities, are meant to care for children as the valuable but vulnerable future of society, while the special care of parents, other whānau, and sometimes even teachers also forges and strengthens affective bonds. Services that appear universal can hence be accepted as part of the normal social order, just as the state provides free education and primary health care for children. But when a service is delivered in a way that marks out that this care *ought* to be the responsibility of someone else—a parent—then services that single some children out—such as the charity-provided "spare" lunches at Tūrama School—become stigmatized care. Children's subsequent engagement with care services at school is therefore the product of an articulation between the state's view of how responsibility for children's care should be distributed and children's own understandings of how care constitutes their status as children and their relationships with adults.

This intersection speaks to the broader questions of this book as, through the particular nature of care services, the neoliberal state provides a structural frame around which children collectively generate meanings and practices according to the particular ways they understand their social position *as children*. This relationship is partly captured in Corsaro's model of interpretive reproduction, whereby children spin spirals of meaning around spokes representing institutional fields (1992, 2015). However, the meanings children make also catch them in their own webs, as they enable and constrain one another's activities: stigma constrains some food options, while ritual enables others. Meanings that enabled younger children to approach the clinic for care become constraints for older children for whom this care is less acceptable. Children's cultural production around responsibility and care therefore form new "structuring structures" (Bourdieu 1984), guiding behaviors, patterning bodies, and contributing to the coproduction of children's health.

In this chapter I begin with an analysis of how children construct care within generational frameworks, before considering how these constructions mediate two kinds of care service at Tūrama School. Through the example of school lunches and other forms of provisioning, I demonstrate how universalized versus selective forms of care are differently understood within children's models of adult-child roles and responsibilities. I then briefly return to the rheumatic fever clinic, introduced in chapter 4, to explore how such generationally structured interpretations of care shift toward adolescence.

Care in Childhood

Issues about care by and for children have been the focus of an extensive body of research in the social sciences. Scholars have largely focused on challenging Western characterizations of children as passive recipients of care by revealing the range and efficacy of children's caregiving practices, how these are unseen or under-acknowledged by adults, and how adults constrain children's care practices in different circumstances (Christensen 1999; Hunleth 2017; Mayall 1993, 1996; Prout 1986; Robson 2004). These debates often center on practical and ethical questions about the appropriate level of children's caregiving and approaches to supporting children's care activities, often by emphasizing children's agency in order to challenge the Western characterizations of children as helpless, incompetent, and vulnerable that often shape policy and practice. Discussions of street children, for example, disrupt expectations about children's capacities to thrive independently of direct adult care (Davies 2008; Gross, Landfried, and Herman 1996; Mizen and Ofosu-Kusi 2013; Panter-Brick 2002); ethnographies of child domestic and paid labor demonstrate the extent of children's economic and social contributions (Kramer 2005; Nieuwenhuys 1996; Reynolds 1991); and accounts of children's caregiving subvert assumptions about the direction of generational care (Andersen 2012; Hunleth 2017; Robson 2004). Likewise, scholars critique the practices of agencies that intend to help children, particularly in developing countries, often based on Western assumptions about childhood (Hecht 1998; Montgomery 2001). The frameworks, agendas, and positions of scholars interested in childhood and care therefore often revolve around tensions between Western discourses of what childhood "should" be and the realities of life for many children around the world, which are not only far from this ideal but appear to be the "choices" of children themselves.

However, the concern with demonstrating children's agency in caregiving has perhaps meant less attention has been paid to how children exercise agency in their receiving of care: the conditions under which children will accept or decline care, the meanings children produce that structure how they negotiate care, and how children's agentive practices mediate the effects of state, institutional, or organizational care on their health. Yet children interact with many forms of biopolitical care that are often subsumed within the public education system, itself a form of state care until transfer of care to legal guardians at the end of the school day. How do children understand, negotiate, and transform those forms of care in the coproduction of their health?

Care, as located in childhood, is grounded in intergenerational processes that shape, as they are shaped by, the help adults and children give to each other. Sociologists interested in the construction of childhood have drawn from Karl Mannheim's (1952) term "generation" to reference the social structure that constitutes children as a distinct social category, analogous to other structured and structuring categories such as class and gender (Alanen 2001; Mayall 2000; Qvortrup 1994). Leena Alanen (2001) analyses how the "generation" category can be both externally defined, for example by age, and, in the Marxist sense, internally constituted in relation to adulthood (analogous to how class is created through the dependent relationship between wage labor and capital). It is in this latter view of childhood, as constructed through intergenerational interactions, that care is implicated as a key mode through which children's status as children is constituted in relation to adults. How care is understood, and the forms that care may take, of course, varies cross-culturally. For example, Jean Hunleth (2017) notes that Zambian children distinguish between Nyanja words for "caring," which translate to protection, help, or advocacy, and "keeping", which typically applies to children but also references anyone perceived as dependent, including the elderly or sick. Thus, an adult may "keep" a child, but not care for them; "keeping" establishes a dependent relationship, child to adult, but "care" creates and maintains interdependent and affective relationships that transcend generations. Children also distinguished between "work," which referred to the domestic or other productive activities they carried out for adults who did not provide material or affective care, and "help," which characterized the exact same activities but only when they reciprocated the "help" children received from adults. Thus, for these Zambian children, "care" is defined by the relationships the activities produce, rather than the intrinsic nature of the activities.

Being a Child

For Tūrama School children, however, adult-child relationships are constructed around the direction of *responsibility* for care—who is meant to care for whom. This concept came up in interviews in which, when I asked, "Who are the people and what are the places that help to keep you healthy?" children's answers focused on adults—particularly mothers, grandparents and aunties—but also fathers, teachers, and Whaea Allison, the "sore throat lady." Children did not name themselves personally, until prompted, and then their contributions were mainly limited to eating fruit. One child named some friends who protected him from bullies. Care, therefore, at least in terms of health, was conceptualized primarily as an adult role.

That adults care for children also became clear when I conducted activities with groups of children asking them to brainstorm "what it means to be a child" and "what it means to be an adult." Children painted a picture of childhood as fun and free, a time when one can "eat lollies" and "don't need to worry." This was a particular type of freedom, because although children saw themselves as free from *responsibility*, they also described a long list of restrictions on what they could do (Can't smoke, can't drink, get told what to do, can't swear. Kids aren't allowed to get girlfriends. Kids are not allowed to drive cars. Can't play violent video games.). Adulthood was described in terms of both responsibilities and freedom from restriction. "Adults have to be more responsible!" one girl contributed to the brainstorm, and another boy thought "[childhood] is better because they don't get to do the hard stuff. Hard jobs." According to the children, adults have to clean, pay the water bill, and "be a mother—you have to bathe them, change their nappies, feed them, buy them clothes, make them a bottle." Adults think, "Man, I wish I never had kids" and "When you grow up as an adult you wish that you were still a kid."

"Do you know," confided one girl, "some people lose their fun, in them? Like they go unfun." This dire picture of adulthood was balanced by the perceived freedoms of adults: "Adults can go out and go to the movies with all our cousins. And they can go out by themself," "Adults get to go with older people, and they get to play on those ticket games, the money- pokies!" "Adults can get jobs!"

Most emergent in these brainstorms was the relationship between children and adults: Children are cared for by adults. Adults are supposed to help children: "When you have a cut they put a plaster on it," "They make sure you're fed," "They love you, care about you," "They give you lots of ice cream," "They get to protect you, look after you." Adults "growl (at children) for not wearing a jumper [sweater] outside during rain."

In contrast to many adult views of childhood, children did not consider themselves to be incompetent—just restricted. One group of boys started phrasing their restrictions in question form, sometimes with answers: "Why isn't children allowed too much sugar? They might get diabetes."

"Why isn't kids allowed to get jobs? Because—kids can't get jobs because—because they're at school. They need to learn first."

"Why ain't children allowed to swear? Because it's naughty words!"

Children also acknowledged their vulnerability, sometimes associating this with their restrictions. Sometimes these vulnerabilities reflected adult fears of violent strangers rather than anything the children had experienced firsthand: "Children are little and we can't go far because we might get robbed or tortured or raped." All groups of children named vulnerabilities they had experienced as part of being a child, such as being bullied or losing family members. "Helpless," one boy explained. "When you're getting a hiding. You're helpless. Especially if it's from your dad."

Vulnerabilities also arose from children's dependency on adults. "If you're young, and your mum and dad die, who would you live with?" asked one boy who had been living with his grandmother.

In this model of childhood, children's lack of power and vulnerability is offset by the net benefits of being cared for by parents and being free from the work and responsibilities of adulthood. This is not to suggest that children did not engage in any caregiving activities. Of course they did, much like the Danish schoolchildren whom Pia Christensen (1999) describes as giving "help":

taking injured peers to the sickroom, fetching items for parents, giving affection, making tea. Some at Tūrama School, like Mila in chapter 7, are placed or place themselves into important caregiving roles for family members. In the Danish context, adults disqualified children's acts of care, particularly in an institution where the mantra was, "If you need help, remember to go and find an adult" (1999, 265), while children themselves gave detailed reports of the ways they helped adults. In the case of Tūrama School, it appears children also conceptualize their caregiving activities as affective "help"; children perform acts of care, but while their autonomy is so restricted, they do not consider themselves to be *responsible* for care. This conceptualization may differ in other contexts where children can carry responsibilities with relative independence. From the Tūrama School children's perspectives, the direction of responsibility is what distinguishes children from adults; hence care given by adults to children both constructs and reflects the natural order of things.

Who Is Responsible for Children's Care?

Notions of responsibility also underpin state discourses of children's care in New Zealand, although the concern here is with establishing just which adults are responsible for children. The neoliberal version of responsibility that couches state views of children's care is a slippery and multifaceted concept, in contemporary definitions, indexing "individual or collective accountability through judgements of one's rational capacities, assessments of legal liabilities and notions of moral blame" (Trnka and Trundle 2017, 4) and connoting agency and autonomy, but also discipline and obligation (Shore 2017). Although the notion of the responsible citizen is not new, in its contemporary form *personal* responsibility represents a key mechanism of neoliberal governmentality (Rose 2007). When applied to health, responsibility discourses enact a form of biopower (Foucault 1990) that mobilizes independent citizens to govern their own bodies using a rhetoric of "personal choice" supported by "health promotion" education rather than government or doctor authority.

This contemporary personal responsibility, as invoked by Minister for Social Development Paula Bennett in the school lunch debate and as understood by parents and teachers, reflects a shift in the past few decades from the historical relationships among individuals, society, and the state in New Zealand. As detailed in chapter 2, social policy in Aotearoa was traditionally based on the accepted principles of the 1930s welfare state, with a wide consensus for a collective responsibility "in order to protect the unfortunate and safeguard the nation's children" (Rice 1996, 483). In the past, the state also took an active role in supporting children's nutrition, including government provision of milk in schools between 1937 and 1967 (New Zealand Milk Board 1978). However, the changing family structures of the 1980s—declining marriage, increasing divorce rates, and a significant rise in single-parent families—led to increased demand on welfare services and spending. The subsequent decline in support for the welfare state among New Zealand people coincided with similar trends in other Western countries and the growing dominance of neoliberal policies: economic deregulation; a reduction and commercialization of state services; and the repositioning of responsibility for well-being with individuals, their families, and the local community (Nairn, Higgins, and Sligo 2012). Within this ideology, children are generally subsumed under the umbrella of familial responsibility (Trnka 2017) and are invoked in powerful discourses that morally frame the good parent as one who "takes responsibility," as seen in the school lunches debate, as well as one who reproduces responsibility by raising responsible citizens.

Yet the neoliberal version of responsibility sits uncomfortably as a framework for lives that are constrained by inequities in power and limited choice, and for children, who cannot be held responsible for themselves. Problems arise when parents do not or *cannot* meet children's needs: when children are coming to school without lunch or suffering from health problems stemming from poverty. A deficit-framed popular discourse of personal responsibility blames parents for causing these issues; meanwhile, what responsibility does society have to the children?

The answer, for New Zealand, has been an uncoordinated patchwork of services to plug the gap. For Tūrama School children without lunch, three services offer alternatives to going hungry. First, neoliberal reform has seen a stepping back of state welfare services in favor of "education" to equip citizens to take responsibility for themselves. Under the mantra of "health promotion," therefore, the 2005 Fruit in Schools program (described in chapter 2) offers free fruit three times a week to children in low-decile schools with a mandate to promote healthy eating (Boyd 2011). Second, the ideology of the welfare state has been replaced with a language of "community empowerment," encouraging local organizations and NGOs to step forward as the state withdraws and placing the decision-making—and the responsibility—for health onto local communities (Cushman 2008). Thus when Labour Party Member of Parliament David Shearer, who put forward the "Feed the Kids" bill, stated that he had changed his thinking and that "each school community should be resourced to find and deliver its own long-term food solutions" (Young 2015), he was likely influenced by this popularized notion of deflecting responsibility back onto communities, leaving the decision-making and implementation of necessary programs to schools, NGOs, and community groups. As part of this community effort, children who come to Tūrama School without lunch have the option of a "spare lunch" provided by charity organization KidsCan (www.kidscan.org.nz). Finally, as part of a global business trend, the socially responsible corporation may claim "responsibility" for helping to combat poverty and thus partially release the state from pressure to intervene. In the case of school lunches, this has taken several forms, including the marketing strategy of catering company Eat My Lunch, which promises to donate a free lunch to a child in need with every lunch purchased (Tūrama School did not take part in this program at the time of my fieldwork), and, on a grander scale, the introduction of the Milk for Schools program by dairy co-operative Fonterra (www.fonterramilkforschools.com).

In theory, these three levels of intervention should mean that every child eats a substantial meal at lunchtime. Yet the efficacy of these services depends on how they are viewed, experienced, and interpreted by children, for whom care takes special meaning in the constitution of identities and relationships. Rather than passive recipients of whatever charity is offered, children actively make meaning around these provisions, which influences when and how they are accepted. Children's nutritional status is therefore a coproduction between the neoliberal governance that shapes their food options and the social meanings and practices that children collectively generate around them.

Pōhara, or "Not Hungry"

There is a distinct dietary pattern across children at Tūrama School. Until they get home from school, standard fare for a child at Tūrama School consists of no breakfast, chips or cookies at lunchtime, a carton of milk, and a piece of fruit.[3] Although this is a typical lunch, there is some variation. Some children, if they have been given money, will buy some hot chips or a pie for breakfast on the way to school. A minority will request a "spare lunch" and receive a sandwich and snack supplied by the KidsCan charity. Parents are more likely to supply younger children with a packed lunch, but often expect the children I worked with, aged eight to twelve, to arrange their own lunch.

This variation may contribute to or reflect some of the different processes through which malnutrition is produced in this context; children's body sizes tend to bifurcate into the very underweight and the very overweight, both manifestations of malnutrition (Ministry of Health 2012; Oliver, Rush, Schluter, et al. 2011; Utter, Scragg, Ni Mhurchu, et al. 2007).

This signature diet comes partly as the result of both deprivation and intervention; as parents struggle to supply lunch for their children, alternatives are offered through school services. However, children translate these services through a lens of adult-child roles and responsibilities, and the resulting social meanings influence which provisions children will tend to accept. Children's nutritional status is therefore not only the product of deprivation and intervention, but their own collective social practices. Children's understandings of poverty, assistance, and adult-child roles mean that while the milk and fruit are typically accepted, most children don't take up the offer of the spare lunch, even when they have little to no food of their own. Instead, most children without lunch will claim they are "not hungry" rather than ask for a spare lunch.

The "spare lunches" provided at Tūrama School consist of a sandwich—usually peanut butter, occasionally jam—on white bread, which is often supplemented with a muesli bar or small packet of nuts as donated stocks allow. The sandwiches are made in bulk, using donated ingredients, by a group of volunteers in the school kitchen every Tuesday, wrapped in cling film and frozen. Each morning, teachers are supposed to ask their class who needs a spare lunch and record the names of those who put up their hands. The numbers are sent to the school office, and the secretary will remove the required number of sandwiches from the freezer, with the expectation that by lunchtime they will have defrosted. The spare lunches are not popular; one child described them to me as "cold bread," and many children claim a distaste for peanut butter[4] (which I capitalized on to avoid sharing my lunch). Staff estimated that they gave out around twenty spare lunches a day, but noted that the number varied; the day before payday more were needed, and some individual teachers would push spare lunches more than others at various times, although this may not have had much effect on how many spare lunches were actually *consumed*.

One morning, while sitting on the mat with a class I had not visited recently, I am surprised when after calling the roll the teacher, Mrs. Charles, instructs the class to go and get their lunches. Some children get up and go immediately to the corridor where their bags are hung, but others hold back, avoiding eye contact. As they return to the circle with their lunches in front of them, I get the sense this has been happening every morning for at least a few days.

As the stamping feet and chatter dies down, Mrs. Charles's voice, quiet and low, cuts across the classroom. "Right. Can you tell Julie why we are doing this?"

"Because you need to have lunch or your brain will fall asleep," one of the girls replies.

"That's right," Mrs. Charles confirms in a sing-song tone. She then proceeds to inspect each child's lunch, one by one. Mila has only a muesli bar, so Mrs. Charles writes her name on the spare lunch order form. "Where's your sandwich, Ruby?" she asks. "You usually have a sandwich. You make it yourself." Ruby, sitting with a packet of chips and an orange (the only piece of fruit in the class), mumbles and avoids eye contact. Many children have only chips or cookies, and so their names are recorded. Five or six children, mostly boys, don't have anything in front of them. Some of them say, "My mum is bringing it later," and Mrs. Charles responds, "I know what that means!" and writes their names down, too.

When the lunch bell rings, a bread bag stuffed with the ordered sandwiches arrives. Mrs. Charles looks at the order form and calls out names. "Mila! Ruby! Kauri! Wiremu! Come and get your lunch!" One or two children come to claim a lunch, but most of the class have already disappeared out of the classroom, leaving Mrs. Charles holding the bag of half-thawed sandwiches.

I watched Mrs. Charles repeat this process a few days later, but she did not continue with it much longer after that, later telling me:

"It got to the stage where I was being the food Nazi, and it got to the stage where I was putting them on the spot, and they would order the spare lunch and then they would just chuck the spare lunch, they would just chuck it away."

While children, when I asked why they did not order a spare lunch, claimed they weren't hungry, in interviews after school I was able to gain more insight.

Twelve-year-old Arya told me that in her class, "hardly anyone gets spare lunch 'cause they're shamed? 'Cause it's like, they're *pōharas* [poor]?" She continues, "Today—someone pranked my name on the spare lunch. And I know, that's not my handwriting."

"Have you ever wanted to get a spare lunch but you haven't because you didn't want people to make fun of you?" I wonder.

"No," says eleven-year-old Nikora, who is with us.

"We always have lunch, aye?" says Arya.

"You always have lunch," I repeat.

"We never, ever, ever—oh well, in term one, 'cause my mum brought like things that, should not be . . . she bought . . . phones, and stuff."

Having established that her lack of lunch had been caused by what she framed as her mother's irresponsible purchasing, Arya goes on to tell me how much her dad gets on payday, which to her is a lot. "I can buy heaps of food if got that much. But they get smokes and that," she laughs, embarrassed, again referring to how her parents spend their money, rather than not having enough. "They could like donate to . . . Save the Child and stuff."

I am not sure what she means, but Arya explains that her mother had donated fifty dollars to buy food for African children.

"But were you saying that in term one you weren't getting the right kind of lunch?"

"Yeah. My—I had . . . to go to school with no lunch." Arya laughs, to show this didn't upset her. "But I never got spare lunch, I just like ate the fruit and that. But in term two, and now, I get money and stuff."

In Patricia Grace's (1986) novel *Potiki*, the Māori people reclaiming their land speak of being, of course pōhara, but also emphatically *not* pōhara, this time referring to the poverty that comes with the cultural death of a people. I understand the word pōhara to connote the indignity and disenfranchisement of poverty, more than just the material state of deprivation, and I suspect it is with this valence that Tūrama School children use the word to signify the absence of something greater than lunch. In this conversation, Arya casts those who get spare lunches as pōhara, but positions herself outside of this category because she always has lunch. Then remembering an earlier time when she didn't have lunch, she blames her mother for irresponsible purchasing, rather than accepting the label of pōhara herself. It is not that her mother did not care, because she never took a spare lunch like those other, pōhara children. Arya then details her parents' finances to show they were definitely not pōhara and tells me about how her parents donate to Save the Children, contrasting her family with the children in Africa who *really* don't have food. Now, she tells me, she always has lunch, because her mother gives her money.

"So do you buy some lunch on the way to school?"

"Yeah. Today I bought some lollies."

To Arya the lollies she buys count as lunch, so she doesn't need to consider a spare lunch, and she clearly isn't pōhara. She continues:

"That's my lunch and . . . and I bought a packet of chips." She tells me her brother stole her chips to give to his friends, and her voice drops, almost to a whisper. "That was for my lunch. That's why I have nothing besides milk and fruit. Oh no, just milk."

Because today was not a fruit day, her lunch has consisted of milk and lollies. Yet this is still a socially acceptable meal. For these children, lunch means more than sustenance; it is also a highly visible symbol of socioeconomic status and of a parent who is giving care as parents should. Because the spare lunches require special—and public— request, this well-intended charity service marks out children who have unfulfilled needs, establishing the idea that lunches are not *meant* to be supplied by the school. Lunches are meant to be supplied by parents. Mrs. Charles's regime of publicly identifying whose parents have and have not supplied them with sufficient lunch, while unusual and short-lived, represents an extreme reinforcement of these social meanings. The unappealing nature of "cold bread" further reinforces this as substandard and therefore stigmatized care. Thus, neoliberal discourses of parental responsibility are translated into the nature of service provision, which children in turn reproduce. Echoing public discourse, children, too, can blame their parents for a failure of responsibility rather than a lack of income.

This invoking of parental irresponsibility appeared in conversations with other children also. In an interview with a group of girls from Mrs. Charles's class, Ngapaea says to Ruby, "You mock Tāmati when he has to get spare lunch." As the girls dissolve into giggles, Ngapaea explains, "She mocks Tāmati when he gets spare lunch. Because he, like, got nearly—he got, like, spare lunch for like a whole term." The girls shriek with giggles.

"Why do you think some children are getting spare lunch?" I ask.

"Because we got a day with no lunch," says Ruby, meaning that she and others sometimes don't have lunch on a given day.

Ngapaea is not willing to claim membership of this group. "Or, their parents, um, are broke."

"Usually they spend it on beers, and cigarettes," adds Alexandra.

Like Arya, the girls here emphasize that getting a spare lunch does not imply a family that has limited economic means but specifically a parent who has misspent their money, prioritizing beers and cigarettes. Also like Arya, the girls position themselves as different from those children. Ruby claims she's never had spare lunch, and Ngapaea admits she had spare lunch when she was younger, but not anymore "because my mum is organized with the lunch."

"Yeah, that's like us," says Ruby. She has forgotten—or is not willing to remember—the two occasions I observed Mrs. Charles ordering her a sandwich after lunch inspection.

"OK, so you always have lunch now. And so now you can just laugh at Tāmati for . . ." the girls giggle. "You guys are so mean!"

"He laughs at us!" Ngapaea protests.

"'Cause we be naughty, like we talk . . ."

"We get in trouble 'cause we talk in class, and then—shame!"

"But, like, when he orders spare lunch we, like . . ." The girls laugh.

Ngapaea finishes, "But he just chucks it away."

In the social meaning collectively understood by children at Tūrama School, asking for a spare lunch designates a child as pōhara. For times when they don't have lunch, then, children have created a range of strategies to negotiate this identity. The most common and socially accepted strategy is to claim they are "not hungry," making choice from necessity (Bourdieu 1984), a state that is not only discursive but may become embodied, as I describe in chapter 6. Some children take a spare lunch and either accept the lower social status that comes with it, or, like Tāmati, throw the lunch away under pressure from teasing. Some children, like Arya and Ngapaea, appropriate the language of responsibility to reframe their lack of lunch as disorganized parenting so as to avoid the pōhara identity. Finally, at times the school receives donations of a food item popular with children, such as fruit cups or packets of trail mix. When this high-value product is included in the spare lunch, some groups of children will collectively decide it is acceptable to order a spare lunch in order to obtain this item. In these circumstances, while the group ostensibly orders a spare lunch solely to eat the chocolate out of the trail mix, it is possible for individuals to make a performance out of picking out the chocolate, and then quietly consume the rest as well.

Possibly the most significant effect of these dynamics, however, is to transform definitions of lunch. When having no lunch designates a child as pōhara, any amount of food, no matter how insubstantial, is enough to be classified as "having lunch," symbolically marking both economic means and a parent's care. The pattern of nutrition at Tūrama School therefore is founded in the one-dollar packets of imported chips and fifty-cent lolly mixes available at the corner store on the way to school.

Milk

The social meanings children ascribe to spare lunches, constituted through notions of who should be supplying the lunch, therefore limit the acceptance and consumption of those lunches. Yet the supplying of food by adults other than parents is not in and of itself interpreted as stigmatized care. Other forms of provisions through school services are taken up with enthusiasm. Children from each class are given the task of collecting the fruit from the Fruit in Schools program three times a week, and the fruit is distributed indiscriminately to everyone at the beginning of break time or eaten together during class time. Likewise, Fonterra's milk has now been knitted into the daily routine of Tūrama School.

The "Milk in Schools" program was initiated in 2012, amid the growing debate about child poverty and the role of government and schools in children's nutrition. Applauded by the government and media alike, Fonterra distributes a free carton of reduced-fat milk to 145,000 children at any primary school that chooses to participate—currently 70 percent of New Zealand's schools ("Fonterra Milk for Schools"). As well as invoking a nostalgia for the historical (state-funded) provision of milk to schoolchildren between 1937 and 1967 (New Zealand Milk Board 1978), the near-universal embracing of the program is probably at least partly because Fonterra, New Zealand's largest company and a national icon of economic success, is owned by 13,000 farmers and is thus emblematic of the idealized, hard-working, tax-paying, rural Kiwi rather than corporate self-interest. Fonterra's justification, as outlined on its website—to give every child "access to dairy nutrition every school day"—does not mention the opportunity to market milk to children, entrenching Fonterra's produce as an institutionalized part of childhoods, or the clear commercial benefit of a generation of children associating milk with nutrition and accustomed to having milk as a daily part of their diet. As milk is marketed as a highly nutritious food, the promotion of this product to children is seen as a socially responsible thing to do—a sentiment reflected in sponsored media coverage (New Zealand Herald 2016).

In contrast to spare lunches, at Tūrama School, nearly all children drink this milk and may even steal or squirrel away additional cartons of milk for later. Thus, milk has in recent times become the staple food of Tūrama School children, largely because of the way it has become embedded in a collective social ritual of consumption.

On a typical day in Mrs. Randall's class, we come into the classroom after morning tea, breathless and sweaty from our soccer game. I claim a spot on the mat with my back against a cupboard, and Cassidee slips in beside me on one side, Caleb on the other. The rest of the children arrange themselves into a circle. Usually when we sit on the mat in Mrs. Randall's class, we sit facing the teacher at the front for instruction. But every day after morning tea the children come in and sit in a circle on the mat. This arrangement is symbolic of milk time, the one time that we can see everyone in the class across the circle.

Mrs. Randall opens the box of milk and hands cartons to the child next to her, who passes them on until the milk has made a full circuit and all of us have one. The cartons are cold, as Mrs. Randall has installed a small fridge in the classroom to keep them in, and some of the boys across the circle hold the cartons against their red cheeks to cool down after soccer.

We shake and puncture our cartons with our straws and sip slowly, prolonging this time of relaxation, because it is a peaceful social time. Today is Whetu's birthday, so Mrs. Randall hands around a container of cookies to celebrate. "You can have one of each kind," she instructs. Some children have brought cookies from home as well, so they can have "milk 'n cookies."

"Miss, can we have our banana now too?" asks Dandre. "So we can have banana milkshakes!" Mrs. Randall laughs, reaching for the basket, and the bananas—the fruit of the day for the Fruit in Schools program—get passed around as well.

Mrs. Randall is drinking a milk too, and she leans back in her chair and chats to Amberlee about her new baby sister. We relax and talk among ourselves, but with mouths full of straws, bananas, and cookies the chatter is not overpowering or loud. Finishing her conversation, Mrs. Randall opens her bookmarked copy of *Matilda* and starts reading aloud.

I sip my milk slowly as I listen. It does not taste bad but is not something I would normally choose to drink. At the start of the year I used to decline the offer of milk and sometimes bring an alternative, but I soon found myself drinking the milk for the pleasure of being included in the group. The milk-drinking ritual brought the class together in companionship and bonding as they are literally and symbolically nurtured by their teacher and one another. The children don't have to drink the milk, but they usually all do. One time, Dandre, upset after being told off, refused to take his milk and his banana. He sat in stony silence while the children around him alternated between drinking their own milk and asking whether he was sure he didn't want any. Usually delighted for "banana milkshake" day, Dandre's rejection was of the social bonding more than of the food, an expression of his upset state.

After we drain our cartons, making sucking noises to get the drops in the corners, we fold them according to the method prescribed by the recycling guidelines. The children taught me how to do this at the beginning of the year, and it took me a couple of tries to learn, but now they say I am very good at it. My carton is always very neat and flat. It requires a bit of technique, but the children are very adept at it, and often a child will ask whether they can do mine. Much like folding origami or paper airplanes, the folding of the cartons is an activity that lets us demonstrate skill, and now we fold juice and other cartons in the same way. One of the boys spills the milk all over himself as he folds the carton. "That's why you're supposed to drink it dry," says Mrs. Randall. A few of the children begin to chant, "Drink it dry, fold it flat, send it back!" Others join in the chorus as we take our folded cartons outside to a special-purpose bin, which will later be emptied and collected by Fonterra for recycling. The cartons are shipped to Thailand to be made into roofing tiles.

This routine is similarly embedded into life in other classrooms. But one day in Mrs. Charles's class, we are sitting in our circle after morning tea, and the children ask, "where's the milk?"

"Where is the milk!" says Mrs. Charles, and she asks one of the children to run and find out where it is. We sit, looking at one another across the circle, waiting. There is a knock at the door, and another teacher puts her head in. "Do you know where the milk is?" she asks. "All my kids are ready for their milk!" As Mrs. Charles gets up to discuss where the glitch in the delivery system may be, I laugh, "This school falls apart when the milk is not delivered, huh?"

"Yeah," says Ruby. "After morning tea we feel like milk, and there's no milk."

This deep routinization of milk drinking—highlighted on the day the milk did not arrive—contrasts with the stigma endured by children who request a spare lunch. Instead, children consume the milk not just because it is provided, but because its universal distribution democratizes its consumption, and because the ritual practices collectively generated by teachers and children together—the circle, the cookies and banana milkshakes, the carton folding—make milk more about the coproduction of a shared social experience of togetherness than nutrition. Spare lunches, which require children to single themselves out and thus indicate difference, poverty, or parental irresponsibility, are less accepted, when chips and lollies, bought cheaply, can symbolically represent material assets and a parent's care.

The pattern of nutrition at lunchtime at Tūrama School therefore is not only a product of deprivation and intervention but also of children's own cultural meanings and social practices, which are collectively produced and directly shape children's bodies in patterned ways. A diet of lollies, bananas, and milk has some nutritional value but is far from balanced and is high in sugar. Furthermore, although a normative discourse of milk as a growth food for children is used as a global marketing strategy (and rarely questioned), Wiley (2007, 2014) argues that the correlations between milk and growth do not represent anything intrinsic to milk, but simply reflect the protein and caloric content of milk—although milk can be a convenient method of delivery. Furthermore, milk comes with its own set of digestive problems. While onset of progressive symptoms for individuals with lactase non-persistence genes typically occurs around adolescence or early adulthood, it is common for children to develop symptoms, in some populations before the age of five (Heyman 2006). Lactose intolerance is common among people of Polynesian ancestry; in a sample of 160 adults with self-reported Māori or Pacific ancestry, 34 percent had the genotype for lactase non-persistence, and the frequency rose with increasing Polynesian ancestry (Roberts, Merriman, and Upton 2010). Yet when the government abdicates responsibility for supplying nutrition, they also leave it in the hands of corporations to decide what form that nutrition will take—a decision that will not be based on objective evaluation of options.

The specific forms that Tūrama School children's food options take there-fore are a product of much wider economic and political circumstances, and par-ticularly ideological notions of how responsibility for children's care should be distributed. Yet children also actively negotiate, accept, or decline these options, based on different moral interpretations of different forms of provisioning. Tūrama School children are not aware that only schools in the poorest commu-nities receive fruit or that for some schools in wealthier areas, the free milk is deemed not worth the program's administrative burden. Because both of these forms of provisioning are universal and routinized, their supply is part of the normal order of things; it is the role of adults in general, including schools and teachers, to care for children. The confluence of neoliberal ideologies of respon-sibility for children's care, and children's own perceptions of the roles of adults, therefore creates the conditions for practices that affect children's health in dis-tinct ways.

Sore Throat Clinic

Thus, the neoliberal version of responsibility comes to shape children's health practices via the particular forms that care services take, contributing to the avoidance of spare lunches in contrast to the uptake of milk. Ideas about the distribution of responsibility also inform the Rheumatic Fever Prevention Pro-gramme, which in turn creates particular experiences that children, again, inter-pret within intergenerational structures.

While neoliberalism has restructured health policy according to notions of personal responsibility, the movement has also transformed the construction and governance of childhood (Tap 2007), making it what Rose calls "the most intensely governed sector of personal existence" (Rose 1999, 123). The surveil-lance medicine that emerged in the early twentieth century targeted the child for intensive monitoring of growth and development through clinics and schools (Armstrong 1995), but neoliberalism has reframed this surveillance in terms of personal—and in the case of children, parental—responsibility for monitoring health.

The way the state views responsibility for rheumatic fever, therefore, means that Tūrama School children still live in poverty but get a clinic, preventive anti-biotic treatment, and a campaign designed to remind their parents to take action for sore throats. An archetypal example of surveillance medicine, the intervention program involves both screening[5] and health promotion and thus brings illness out of the hospital and into community life, constituted as a con-stant risk to be monitored but conceptualized, prevented, and treated at the level of the individual family. Responsibility for preventing rheumatic fever is placed on the shoulders of families, starting with media campaigns urging parents to take their child to the doctor for a sore throat. "If we got it checked earlier, he wouldn't have this," a young boy says in the television advertisement, pointing to his brother's scar. "If I knew that this sickness started with a sore throat, I would have taken him to the doctor earlier," says his mother in another advert. "It's not cool to take the risk of 'I'll see if it's okay tomorrow.' As soon as your kid gets a sore throat, you need to get it checked," warns the mother of another young boy. These statements, coupled with horrified descriptions of having a child in hospital and seeing the child almost die, give the implicit message that the family is responsible for rheumatic fever prevention. There is no mention of the fact that between one-third and two-thirds of acute rheumatic fever cases are not preceded with a known sore throat event (Robin, Mills, Tuck, et al. 2013; Veasy, Wiedmeier, Orsmond, et al. 1987) or that children themselves may not recognize or report their sore throats. The framing of rheumatic fever prevention does not recognize how impractical it may be for families with multiple children and working parents to take children to a doctor for every sore throat—although this issue is at least partly solved for communities with school clinics—or that outbreaks of rheumatic fever might point to hazardous socioeconomic inequality and be better addressed through economic policy. The illness is characterized as an individual problem, the solution is for families to monitor and medicate their children, and the school clinic is established to support parents and children to deal with their problem. Thus, out of ideas about responsibility, rheumatic fever enters the lives of all children at Tūrama School to stamp their bodies with antibiotics, anxiety, and hypervigilance of the throat—an embodiment of surveillance that I explore in chapter 6. Here, I consider the way this state conceptualization sits alongside children's views on responsibility for care, shaping the way that children accept with enthusiasm, avoid, or negotiate care from the clinic.

In many ways, the integration of the sore throat clinic into Tūrama School has had positive effects. As I described in chapter 4, large numbers of children access care from the clinic on a regular basis and have a good experience of health care that may translate to a positive view of external health-care services as well. Although primarily serving as a sore throat and skin infection clinic, Whaea Allison and Deb do identify and treat or refer children for other illnesses on an ad hoc basis. Children's enthusiasm, however, drops off as they graduate to the combined year seven/eight class, for ages eleven to thirteen. Whaea Allison had to make special effort to make sure these older children—particularly the year eights—were checked regularly. The clinic therefore works very well for children but less well for adolescents.

From the perspectives of children, the clinic is not stigmatized care; like the milk, the clinic intervention is universal—every child is checked under the throat-swabbing program, not just those whose parents cannot get them to a

doctor. The clinic system also fits with children's own model of childhood, reinforcing the adult-child relationship of care. For children, adult monitoring of
their health status is a normal care practice that establishes adult and child identities. Surveillance medicine, therefore, is another form of adult governance
over children's lives (Rose 1999) that this generation has grown up experiencing
as the normal order of things. Teachers ask children if they have a sore throat in
the same way that mothers check on children's health. Whaea Allison is warm,
motherly, and affirming and takes children through a diagnostic process that is
translated into a practice of care. Ten-year-old Tupono describes this process in
great detail for me:

"First of all you stand on the scales. They check your weight. And, sometimes
that could do with sore—like, a illness you can put on heaps of weight or you
could lose heaps of weight? And . . . so I stayed the same, oh—thirty to thirty-
four? A lot less than everybody in my class and . . . then next they get you to check
your temperature and your ear with the ear temperature thingy. What is it called?
It's a m . . . Do you know what it's called?"

"Thermometer?" I supply.

"Oh, yeah," Tupono continues. "I knew it had 'meter' at the end. Then they
get this, so you know those things that you get your ear wax out, those pokey
things, they have a long one but not double sided, they stick it in your mouth
and they put it in this jar to keep it clean while they deliver to the doctors. And
that's it."

Through this process, children understand Whaea Allison to be assessing
their sickness, and in doing so she is showing care and protecting them from
the dangers of disease. Tupono, a bright boy with a particular interest in medicine that he has acquired through reading medical literature in church, gave
the most technical description of the clinic processes of all the children I talked
to, including an interpretation of why he was being weighed. Children were
actually weighed to determine the dosage of antibiotics but often took careful
notes of their measurement and connected this with the monitoring of their
health and development: ten-year-old Ngawaina imagines Whaea Allison weighs
her "to see how big I've grown." Meanwhile, some children mistook Allison's
assessments for treatment. I observed a young girl, after being swabbed, saying
she still felt sick, and Allison gently explained, twice, checking for understanding, that the swab is a test, not a treatment. When she was not made aware that
children thought they were seeking treatment, Allison was not able to clarify.
Ten-year-old Anton, a regular visitor to the clinic, described how he would feel
better and his cough would be gone for the rest of the day after being checked
at the clinic; he understood "sore throat" to mean "coughing and fevers" and
connected the abatement of his cough with being swabbed. He did note that the
cough would be back the next day though, but he was only allowed to go to the
clinic one day every week:

". . . If I get checked, like, my coughs is gone, for, like, the whole day? And then after the other day, I can't go to the sore throat lady, because you only allowed one day, and then . . . it just comes back."

Hence, children's experience of the clinic processes matches and reinforces their concept of adulthood and childhood, that children are cared for and protected by adults. Children may come to the clinic seeking the care and approval of Whaea Allison as much as to have a sore throat checked.

For older children, however, these dynamics can have the opposite effect. Children in the combined year seven/eight class, aged eleven to thirteen, presented less often to the clinic than those in years five and six; the older children drag their feet to avoid class checks, and Whaea Allison must make a special point of tracking these children down. This form of surveillance medicine, configured around adult-child dichotomies, is welcomed by those who embrace their child status but resisted by older children who see themselves transitioning toward adulthood and anticipate adult relations with health professionals in negotiating their care. The clinic procedures, however, position them squarely as children. At a time when young adolescents are claiming their bodily autonomy, the clinic requires them to hand their bodies over to an adult to be weighed, inspected, felt, and inserted with thermometers and swabs. The public nature of the clinic's work, which younger children capitalized on as an opportunity for social interaction, became an embarrassing intrusion into privacy for older children. Sometimes older children would instead visit the clinic quietly at lunchtime, when their check could be made discreetly and in private. Furthermore, even the year six girls had begun to become self-conscious about being weighed: "Today my weight was fifty-one," Ngawaina whispered to me in our interview. "I gained heaps of weight." By year seven or eight, for many girls, in particular, weight is no longer positively associated with growth, and the process of being weighed puts them into a vulnerable and embarrassing position.

Children's engagement with care services is therefore mediated by their conceptions of adulthood and childhood and how their perceive their own status within this binary. In a model in which childhood is established in relation to adulthood, the shifting and liminal stage of adolescence makes for unstable identities within a framework of adult authority and child vulnerability, adult care and child help. These young people often still want or need care; they are still disturbed or frightened by the rheumatic fever campaign, and some do negotiate their own path to the clinic's care. Despite its common association with childhood, they still drink their milk together, long limbs sprawled on the mat, while their teacher reads them Māori myths from a picture book. But the children who in year six were still taking a spare lunch never do in year seven and eight, and their teacher does not bother asking anymore. These are young people at the beginning of what will be a long period of in-between-ness, navigating generational structures of care in a society also not sure whether they are children or adults either, and this structural awkwardness will also remodel the patterns of their health care and practices.

Conclusion

Three years after the day I sat with children arguing over my lunch, a new organisation initiated a campaign calling for the government to supply all New Zealand school children with lunch. The Eat Right, Be Bright campaign (www .eatrightbebright.org.nz) draws on the language of children's rights to argue against ideologies of parental responsibility, while pointing to successful programs overseas that show that uptake of school lunches is high, stigma is reduced, and health benefits are enjoyed by children of all economic backgrounds when nutritious, appealing meals are supplied to everyone. A concurrent media article (Nikula 2018) calculated an annual cost of $720 million based on the well-established and comprehensive Finnish model. Still, the New Zealand government has rejected far more modest proposals targeting primary-school aged children at low-decile schools that budget $3.4–$14 million per year.

State policy on this issue, therefore, is not so much a matter of economics as it is of ideology. The services supplying provisions and health care to Tūrama School are, directly or indirectly, the products of neoliberal state views on responsibility for children's care, whether the service is a free fruit program wrapped in health promotion, or a service provided by a corporation capitalizing on the vacuum created by the state's abdication. In passing off this issue to NGOs and corporations, however, the state also vacates the possibility of care that is child-centered, coordinated, and adequately resourced to alleviate the issues arising from poverty. KidsCan does not have the funds or infrastructure to offer an appealing and universal lunch, while Fonterra has little motivation to supply a nondairy substitute for lactose-intolerant children who may be equally in need of calories and protein. The rheumatic fever clinic, operating under a small and specific community contract, can refer families for housing support only under tight criteria, while accountability for the structural conditions underlying children's poverty and ill health remains contested.

The nature of these services, though, is not wholly determined by adults, because they are interpreted by children who hold their own, different ideas about what responsibility for care means. From children's perspectives, care given by adults and *society* is part of what constitutes childhood. The degree to which these services operate in congruence with children's generational understandings of care therefore shapes how children bring these services to life and transform them through social activity. Children collectively make spare lunches into stigmatized care, while, together with teachers, they generate ritualized practices of consumption from the milk and fruit that are supplied to everyone. Younger children enjoy their status-affirming care from Whaea Allison but those transitioning into adolescence experience friction when this care reaffirms their status as children and consequently form new patterns of engagement. Thus, children make culture within the structures created by society, but these cultural meanings and practices also, in the Geertzian sense, constrain children in their own webs of meaning, structuring one another's future practice. Children's care, and subsequent health effects, are a form of coproduction between the neoliberal state and the practices of children who interpret care within generational frameworks.

6

Embodying Inequality

Life for many children at Tūrama School involves coping with bodies that never quite seem to have enough of everything they need: food, sleep, warmth. In winter, particularly, I watched bodies shiver or withdraw, yawn and sneeze, the tactical, homeostatic responses of systems trying to compensate for physiological and psychosocial stressors. Yet their conditions—poverty, institutional structures, even the climate—also seemed to restructure children's bodies in deeper ways, hinting at habituated modes of adjusting to chronically suboptimal environments when there is little else that can be done. Bodies that shiver and emote and feel pain are functioning as they should, but bodies that do not perceive hunger when they have no food, that are not anxious under threat, or that are numb to the cold, have learned to accommodate enduring conditions they cannot change.

My analysis of these habituated bodies comes at a time in childhood studies when, after a turn toward the socially constructed nature of childhood, the body has re-emerged as a focus of children's lived experience: both how the body structures children's social experience (by size, shape, age, gender, and so on) and the ways in which the social world structures children's bodies (civilizing, regulating, and disciplining) (Hörschelmann and Colls 2009; James 1993; Mayall 1996; Prout 2000b). Increasingly, this line of childhood research has followed Prout (2000a, 2005) in viewing the body as neither essentialized nor separate from the social, but as the material foundation of children's social experience and produced in concert with the social. Already central to children's lives, the body is especially implicated in the study of health and illness, with health-care practices often performed in response to experiences of the body—symptoms, sensations, emotions—and thus reliant on "reading" and interpreting bodily signals. Yet these experiences are not universal or standard but are patterned by local social context through embodied learning and the cementing of practices over time—the forming of habituated bodies.

An understanding of children's health, therefore, must begin with an understanding of the processes that shape how children may come to experience their bodies differently in different contexts. The literature concerned with embodied childhood has long recognized the way that schools, in particular, regulate children's behavioral, cognitive, and emotional development (Christensen 1999; Christensen, James, and Jenks 2001; Mayall 1996, 1998, 2002, 2015; Prendergast 2000; Prendergast and Forrest 1998). This research reveals the power structures embedded in the way adults constrain and shape children's bodies, and the role of children's agency in this negotiation, but tends to stop short of a detailed biosocial analysis, with less attention to the specific processes of the body that are implicated and how these feed back into the social experience. Parallel research in biological anthropology picks up where the social research left off, diving under the skin to trace how different structural environments manifest in distinct biological signatures (e.g., Flinn 2011; Panter-Brick, Todd, and Baker 1996), but tends to position children as passive absorbers of their environment, omitting the interpretive elements of bodily experience that make this a dialectical process.

This chapter aims to bring these two literatures a step closer together, by considering the biosocial production of the experience of the body, with a focus on how children's internal perceptions of their body are socially calibrated. Using the examples of temperature, hunger, and sore throat, I unpack the processes through which children coproduce their bodies at the intersection of local resource distribution and both adult and child cultures, in the overlapping fields of home and school. I argue that bodily perceptions are biosocially learned and accommodated, becoming part of the habitual practices of the self, and that these experiences, and their subsequent health-care practices, can be implicated in the production of unequal bodies. Children not only learn to interpret their bodily perceptions in culturally mediated ways, but this learnt process in turn structures the perception and experience of the body, shaping bodily practices, and coproducing the biosocial body itself.

The "Reembodiment" of Childhood

After a major shift in attention toward the socially constructed nature of childhood, the turn of the twentieth century saw a "reembodiment" of childhood research coinciding with renewed interest in the body in social theory more generally (Prout 2000a). While previous research focused on embedded power structures and the significance of the discursive to children's experience of the body, some authors (Colls and Hörschelmann 2009; Prout 2000a, 2005) have challenged the "disembodiment" of childhood, critiquing the implicit Cartesian dualism reproduced in a focus limited to how bodies are socially produced and experienced. In particular, Alan Prout has expanded upon Shilling's notion of the body as "unfinished" in relation to childhood. In his (2000b) edited volume, researchers from social anthropology and sociology took up an approach to embodied childhoods that views the biological and social bodies working in synthesis to model and remodel each other over the course of the life span. While children have long been considered incomplete versions of adults, this notion that adult bodies also are unfinished has sparked more serious consideration of the processes through which the social and physical bodies develop dialectically, rather than through fixed, distinct stages of biological development (Worthman 1993). This thinking parallels a shift in biological anthropology, which likewise saw increased attention to the ways that the social environment becomes embodied in the development and microprocesses of the body, shaping trajectories of growth and patterns of morbidity and mortality (e.g., Panter-Brick 1998b).

Under this paradigm, researchers working at the nexus of medical anthropology/sociology and childhood have examined how the body is implicated in the lived experience of childhood through the embodiment of social relations— that is, the way that the body forms the basis for social relations and so shapes and codifies, while in turn being shaped and codified by, the social world. Key markers of the body include age, used particularly by school institutions to designate status (by academic class), and body size, which constitutes standards of normalness and difference both for medical professionals and for children in peer cultures (James 1993, 2000). In this way, the body mediates social experience; children have variable subjective experiences of the social world according to how they look and behave in comparison to their peers, and individuals' experiences change as their bodies do.

Yet while the social is grounded in the materiality of the body—its size, shape, performance, gender, and appearance (James 1993)—the social experience also mediates the body. In addition to shaping the body itself, social expectations and experiences also influence how children learn to be in their bodies, as seen through comportment, behavior, emotions, sensation, and health. A main focus of this literature has been the institutional environment, where health practices are structured according to the agenda of teachers and the formal curriculum, in contrast to the home environment, where children have much more autonomy in their health-care practices (Mayall 1996). Authors have drawn from Bourdieu's habitus (1984; 1977) or Elias's concept of civilizing the body (1978, 1982) to theorize the processes through which the school environment initially becomes embodied and to emphasize how these habitual practices linger in the body long after school has ended. This literature examines the way in which the school regulates, civilizes, or disciplines bodies (Mayall 2002; Valentine 2009), in addition or contrast to the socialization that occurs at home, and with the focus on the way embedded power structures enable adults to shape children's bodies and restrict their bodily autonomy. The institutional environment also uses disciplinary techniques to compel children to subdue or control their bodies, including shaming and punishment. Those better able to habituate their bodies appropriately to fit the school are less likely to be on the receiving end of disciplining tactics or social stigma. For example, Christensen, James, and Jenks argue that children's bodies, disciplined to "eat, sleep, wash and excrete, mostly, at specific and regular times" (2001, 208) internalize and become patterned by the temporal structures of the day. This is not a one-sided process, however, as children's agency plays a role in this interaction. While bodily discipline is promoted by teachers who require children to sit still and work quietly, by deliberately adopting the correct bodily posture and appearance—for example, by pretending to look for a book off the shelf, or bending the head over a page—children can strategically "pass off" whispering to friends or taking time for oneself as "work." Hence, as much as schools shape bodies, children also play a major role in the coproduction of their own bodies by acting within and responding to the structures of school.

Such behavioral modifications are often not temporary but become absorbed into the habitus and migrate across fields, interpolating the home habitus as well (Mayall 2015). While the influence of schools on children's bodies can be considered as benign or pastoral (Christensen, James, and Jenks 2001), and certainly it can be useful for children to regulate their bodies for other contexts, this line of research reveals how school can be taken for granted as a powerful mediator of child—and eventually adult—bodies. However, these analyses tend to stop short of a deeper unpacking of the dialectic between the social and the biological processes of the body, which could extend understandings of how the social environment shapes embodiment. Institutions such as schools structure the way that children learn to read and interpret their bodies in quite fundamental ways, and in some circumstances this may contribute to human variation and less benign disparities between children.

In biological anthropology, research has shown how social conditions interact with biological processes to produce differently embodied childhoods. Working with children in the Caribbean, Mark Flinn shows how family structure and events can alter cortisol profiles, which directly contribute to illness events (Flinn 1999; Flinn and England 1995, 1997; Flinn, Ward, and Noone 2005). Similarly, Catherine Panter-Brick shows how the diverse social living conditions of homeless, rural and urban dwelling children in Nepal impact stress responses (Panter-Brick and Pollard 1999) and growth (Panter-Brick, Todd, and Baker 1996). Such research reveals just how deeply the social environment is woven into the microprocesses of the body. However, the quantitative nature of this research tends to collapse the social into broad categories—for example, "street children" versus "school children" (Panter-Brick, Todd, and Baker 1996). So, on the one hand, the embodiment literature from social anthropology and sociology unravels the role of the interpretive and the structural in children's embodiment, while the biological literature teases out the microprocesses that are biosocially shaped underneath the skin. My hope here is to bring these two literatures a step closer together by extending consideration of bodily processes within an interpretive framework.

This perspective can be seen in the issue of children's toileting practices. Scholars have described the authority of U.K. schools over children's toilet access, illustrating how children's self-care practices at home contrast with their lack of autonomy at school (Mayall 1996, 1998; Prendergast 2000). Invoking a children's rights discourse, this literature documents toileting at school as a source of discomfort, shame, or distress, especially for children who are still developing this technique of the body; Prendergast (2000) describes children being refused access to the toilet, and the embarrassing situations that could arise when children wet or menstruated through their clothing. Poor sanitary conditions and perceptions of safety and security of school bathrooms can also cause children to avoid going to the toilet at school (Lundblad and Hellström 2005).

However, re-centering the body shows that the control of schools over children's toileting practices is more than an issue of rights or emotional well-being. Prendergast (2000) unpacks the effects of school on the body in this regard most thoroughly, describing a "weighty mindfulness" of menstruation burdening girls across U.K. schools: girls must be constantly and completely mindful of this process of the body, having to predict, prepare for, negotiate, and protect their periods, with strong social sanctions and stigmatization befalling any girl who fails to manage her period unobtrusively. However, from here questions emerge about the processes through which the biological body and the social become intertwined: How does this mindfulness affect the way girls learn to "be" in their bodies, their perception of the signs of impending menstruation, and possibly the subsequent construction of premenstrual syndrome?[1] Likewise, for children in schools where toileting is closely controlled, quite complex bodily processes—taken for granted by adults—are asked of them. Children are required to predict when they might need to go to the toilet in future and go to the toilet *before* the urge is strongly felt. This requires a "tuning in" of attention to the signs of particular parts of the body, in order to remember to check in with and notice subtle sensations indicating the state of one's bladder, *at particular times or in particular spaces.*[2] This represents a way in which children's bodies structure the social—shaping teachers' and children's practice—but also of how the social shapes the processes of the body. As children learn to become attuned to these particular signals of the body, they develop a practice of perceiving the body: a synthesis of the body's biological signals structured by the social (in this case temporally and spatially) that become cemented into the physical self.

Toileting restrictions may also have health effects; evidence suggests that limiting access to the bathroom may alter bladder and sphincter function and is considered a factor mediating the development or persistence of urinary tract infections and other issues (Cooper, Abousally, Austin, et al. 2003). Thus, a closer focus on the particularities of body-social relationships shows how the institutional world of the school shapes children's bodies in very fundamental ways, in the internal calibration of attunement to and interpretation of bodily signals that may have further implications for health, as well as psychosocial well-being. My aim in this chapter therefore is to push the analysis of the body further within this literature, via more detailed examination of the biosocial microprocesses that solidify into variation in ways of being in the body that can germinate variable patterns of health.

Bourdieu and the Body

Regulation, body work, and other such practices of the body, shaped by local concepts of what bodies should be in a given context, solidify over time into the *habitus*, meaning that children who have experienced similar social conditions embody these in similar ways. As described in chapter 1, Bourdieu's concept of habitus refers to a "structuring structure" (Bourdieu 1984, 170): the way that people come to embody their social environment through routinized participation in structured social systems that predispose them to perceive, think and feel— or "taste"—in culturally guided ways. Thus, bodily practices are the reproduction (and reinforcement) of those culturally patterned tastes, which then shape the way the world is perceived.

Such bioculturally constituted practices shape not only perception of the world, but perception of the body itself. A useful concept from phenomenology is Husserl's (1962) notion of intentionality, or the "toward-which" orientation of our being in the world. As Desjarlais and Throop eloquently put it, "central to the temporal and embodied structure of human experience is the existential fact that we are emplaced in a world that always outstrips the expanse of our being" (2011, 90). Given a world that is far greater than our ability to experience it, we can focus only on limited aspects—a conditioning of experiential focus that calcifies into a culturally patterned habitus. Likewise, even the body itself, at any given time, provides far greater an expanse of internal information than our attention can hold. We notice different aspects of our bodies at different times, and as we tune in to one part—aching shoulders, thirsty throat, anxious breathing—other sensations recede into the background. This is what Csordas terms "somatic modes of attention" or "culturally elaborated ways of attending to and with one's body in surroundings that include the embodied presence of others" (1993, 138). As illustrated by the example of toileting in schools earlier, which aspect we "tune into" and when, and how frequently we do so, are at least partially socially ordered. Children are socialized to tune into their toileting needs according to temporal and spatial cues (break times and spaces). We are more likely to notice hunger at socially designated mealtimes, we tune into pain when describing it to a doctor, and we can have attention diverted away from the body entirely during captivating social events.

Importantly, the social ordering of the body shapes the interpretation of and response to those perceptions, with implications for health: hunger perception helps to shape nutritional intake; temperature perception protects the body from homeostatic stress; and pain perception has a range of health implications, including for social and medical aspects of health care. Moreover, as Bourdieu notes, the habitus does not only organize practices and perception but is also a "structured structure" (1984, 170) where distinctive modes of being are internalized and reproduced within social classes. The examples I explore in this chapter are particular to a social group whose experiences are typified by poverty and social marginalization, and whose sensory modes therefore represent the perpetuation of an embodiment of social inequality. Finally, the structuring of the senses that occurs in early life may set trajectories of bodily experience and response that continue into adulthood, long after the childhood environment has changed.

I emphasize the generative capacity of Bourdieu's concept, taking habitus as an open and malleable structuring structure that guides, or disposes, but does not determine the course of biosocial development and that shifts, mutates, and opens up new gaps where subcultures can emerge. As illustrated in the previous chapter, children's peer cultures are important here; children produce their own field of structures, which are distinct from adults' but operating at a higher gear of revolution, rapidly mutating to evolve new structural forms as children acquire new information and experience. Often overlooked as a serious force structuring children's embodiment, as this chapter will show, the intersection of children's cultures with institutional structures and resource constraints can shape a suite of practices that then become embodied—in this case, through a modeling of perception.

The Body as Barometer

A challenge of bodily ethnography is in knowing another's experience of the body when that experience can only be understood in reference to oneself. As such, a great deal of this chapter is speculative, composed of scraps of evidence that hint at a different experience of the body. I cannot really assess what children are feeling. However, in drawing from my experience of my body as a form of data, I follow in the tradition of sensory ethnographers like Robert Desjarlais and Loïc Wacquant who engage in "participant sensation" (as opposed to observation) or "feeling along with" to reveal new perceptory orientations (Howes 2006). Desjarlais (1992) uses his bodily experience to access an understanding of shamanic rituals, while acknowledging the limitations of his ability to truly experience his body in the same way the Nepalese healer to whom he was an apprentice did. Instead, through comparisons of his experience with reported experiences of the healer, Dejarlais conceptualizes a hybrid form of embodied experience, recognizing that his body and its perceptions are founded in his previous life experience and that those continue to shape his experience of the shamanic world. In his ethnography of boxing in inner-city Chicago, Wacquant (2004) documents the changes that occur in his body in parallel to his observations about the bodies of the men training alongside him. Although his background was quite different from that of his informants in the gym, the comparison of the changes in his body to the bodies of other boxers at different stages of development—the ontogenesis of rhythm, stamina, and bodily discipline produced by social rules and cultural norms—verified the generalizability of the personal. Through this process of pedantic autophenomenology in reference to their "native" peers, both authors could triangulate their experiences and gain insight into these specific ways of being in the body.

However, although researchers working with adults can access detailed descriptions of how others experience their bodies, this access becomes more difficult with children, who are less experienced at translating their embodied knowledge into verbal expressions. My methodology here therefore relies heavily on observation—noticing the times when my perceptions of my body seemed out of synchronicity with how the children were experiencing the same environment—and comparison of my experience with the experience of other adults.

It was common for me to use my perceptions in a different way from the children I worked with; through my additional years of schooling I had developed a trained ear for the voice of the teacher, an eye for spelling errors, and an inner sense of when teachers were looking and when they were not. The school environment catalyzed a reawakening of habitus-past and, like riding a bicycle, that sense of "how to be" quickly returned. I was less at ease on the playground, where the physical growth since I was at primary school meant that my body was now out of sync with my internal sense of what I could do. I could remember how it would feel to swing around the bars and turn cartwheels, and felt how to do it in my body, but in the time since I had been an avid practitioner of the jungle gym I had lost strength and flexibility, while the physics had changed as my body matured. I was left with the embodied memory of my ten-year-old self, a knowledge that was no longer applicable in a thirty-year-old body (I learned this the hard way—falling on my head). Despite some prior experience, I also did not have close to the same sense of rhythmic coordination to swing poi[3] that many girls at Tūrama School had developed. These were all understandable differences between what my body was habituated to and what the children did with their bodies, products of different developmental stages, experience, and cultural activities. However, there were two recurring times when I was particularly disconcerted by an apparent difference in experience—two forms of bodily perception that I hadn't considered might be so culturally learned. These involved thermoregulation—particularly feeling the cold—and perceptions of hunger.

"Their Thermostat Is Not Working Properly": Perceiving the Cold

A cavalier attitude toward the cold is a cultural feature of Aotearoa, and it is not uncommon to see even adults wearing minimal clothing and footwear in winter. However, in this region of South Auckland, the temperature drops to an average low of 10°C in July and can fall as low as 0°C overnight. In a microclimate created by surrounding mountain ranges, on winter mornings I would often drive down the motorway south and watch the thermometer drop a degree or two as I neared the town where Tūrama School was located.

On a Monday in July, I leave a trail of dark footprints across the frosted grass as I walk into school, and wrapped up in a wool scarf, hat, and jacket, I sit down on the hard gymnasium floor for assembly, shivering against the cold surface. "It's so cold!" I moan.

"It's not cold," the girls next to me say. Some of them are wearing sweatshirts, but many are in only a T-shirt. I am wearing four layers.

"Yes, it is!" I argue. "I bet it's one degree." I look up the temperature on my phone, and it is 10°C, and I pout, "well, it's still *really* cold."

Meanwhile, Mrs. Randall sits on a chair overseeing the two lines of children in her class sitting on the floor. "Whetu," she says, "take that jumper [sweatshirt] off. It's not school uniform." The principal is "cracking down" on correct uniform, she says. Whetu complies, and shivers, stretching his T-shirt up to his chin and hunching over. "I'm going to get sick," he mumbles, although his hacking cough suggests he already is.

In general, children of Tūrama School tended to be underclothed in winter, and the striking contrast between how scantily dressed they were and my many layers of clothing was matched only by the contrast in how much we were bothered by the cold. While I would complain about the cold—in part attempting to make conversation—the children rarely did, and instead, as happened in the gym, would disagree with my assessment of the temperature. However, there were times when the children did feel the cold—Whetu, for example, noticed the difference when he was made to remove his sweatshirt. Inside the classroom, children would huddle against the weak heaters that lined the wall next to the mat. In another class, boys in T-shirts and shorts would drape themselves in blankets and shuffle around like old men. One class had collected a large number of goods for a secondhand stall for the school fair, and after the event, children were allowed to claim unsold items to take home. The objects of most intense negotiation were four large oil heaters, reserved with names written on sticky notes. At the end of the day I watched the lucky children bending over backward, hugging their prize to their chests as they walked off home to families who probably couldn't afford the power bill to run them.

Yet much of the time, I felt like I was on a different planet—one where frost and wind and rain were a misery unless properly buffered with wool hats, thick socks, and a warm jacket. I—like the teachers—wore sheepskin boots and a knitted scarf, and I was *still* cold. Yet children dressed in T-shirts and shoes with holes in them shrugged when I said it was cold. It was not that they didn't ever feel cold; it was that their threshold for intolerable cold seemed a lot higher than mine.

I was not alone in the sense that I was experiencing a different environment. Mrs. Charles, too, described her own sense that the children's perception of their body temperature was underdeveloped when she found herself instructing children to remove clothing because they were too hot.

She tells me: "Mila today was wearing her sweatshirt, which wasn't a school one, and she was wearing her black jacket at lunch time, and she was sweating, and she had a sore head, and she had sore legs. And I said 'Take your jacket off and take your sweatshirt off and go and have a drink.' And she did all that and then she came back and said 'I feel much better.'"

Mrs. Charles continues: "I didn't think she needed her sweatshirt on today because it was hot, but she just, 'Oh, I'm cold.' I said, 'But it's not cold.' I said, 'Here I am walking around [in a sleeveless shirt]' and, yeah, she was hot and she was sweating . . . . So I think that's got a little bit to do with it. Their thermostat is not working properly."

Meanwhile, parental discourse about their children's illness was saturated with descriptions of the struggle to keep their children warm. Mothers battled on two fronts, fighting not only to keep cold weather from infiltrating poor housing but also fighting their children to keep them sufficiently clothed. Te Paea attributed ten-year-old Tupono's three bouts of strep throat to the cold winter, describing how the two of them would sleep in their living room "because it's easier to cordon off and keep warm" but that Tupono would throw off his clothes when he warmed up, "then he'll get up and go to the toilet and he'll get a chill."

Adrienne, having finally got the Housing New Zealand house she needed for her family, described the efforts she made to keep them warm in a house that was still "frickin' freezing like hell, like I go through a lot of power, aye, 'cause I'm trying to keep the house warm for them."

"And then they wear a singlet!" I laugh, gesturing at bare-armed Victor.

Likewise, Aranui described her exasperated attempts to keep her ten-year-old son Wiremu warm to prevent him getting sick with asthma: "It would be the no clothes, playing outside with his sister, yeah, so they'd both be out in this cold air. And I'd be walking round going, 'Put some clothes on like I told you, stay inside,' but I have to keep them physically inside."

Aranui also found herself up at three or four in the morning piling blankets on her children who were coughing and "curling up" but had not realized they were cold.

It seemed that I was not alone in finding I noticed the cold—or the heat—while children did not. Instead, children in general were still developing their ability to perceive and respond to environmental or thermoregulatory signals, while parents actively compensated for and socialized their children to notice the cold and stay indoors or dress more warmly. Teachers also stepped into this role on occasion, but because children at school generally did not have additional clothing to put on, teachers tended not to say anything when children were under-clothed. However, Mrs. Charles, who claimed to take on a "mother hen" role as a teacher, described in an interview with me how she would tell children to warm up or take clothes off to cool down, explaining: "A lot of my kids will have to be told to take their sweatshirts off, take their jackets off. They have no idea of just doing it because their body is being regulated and things temperature-wise . . . And like I said before, I can't teach them anything. They are not able to learn if their body temperature is not right and they are hungry. Quite often I tell them go and put a sweatshirt on or go and sit by the heater. I don't mind if they are wearing a pink sweatshirt to school, just make sure [the principal or deputy principal] don't see it."

Described here, therefore, is a process of drawing children's attention to their bodies and instructing them on how to regulate their temperature: a socialization of bodily perception. This implies that children do not innately know how to notice their discomfort, recognize their body temperature as the source of this discomfort, or understand the correlation with the environmental conditions in the same way as adults. Instead, children must learn this as part of a wider process of learning to be in their body. With a deluge of sensory information coming from both inside and outside of the body, far more than can possibly be perceived at one time, children learn which signals to tune into and which to tune out in ways that are culturally patterned. In Aotearoa, where attitudes toward the cold can be more relaxed and children may be socialized (by peers as well as adults) toward "toughness," the patterning of children's experience of body temperature may already look quite different from that of children in other places. At Tūrama School, the convergence of institutional regulations and poverty create another permutation in this patterning, which reinforces the structuring of bodily perception.

Constraints on Warm: Tuning Out the Cold

The way that the parents draw children's attention to the temperature of the environment and related temperature of the body is an example of classic socialization of how to be in a body, similar to, for example, Geurts's (2003) description of Anlo-Ewe socialization toward balance. However, in the example of children at Tūrama School, I argue that children's learned perception of their bodies is not only shaped by adult socialization. While children are still learning to notice the cold, in this environment their lack of power and submissive status to adult authority constrains their ability to respond, even if they are tuned into these bodily or environmental signals. I suggest that when children do not have the capacity to respond to perceptions of cold or hunger, then the sensitivity of their attunement toward these perceptions may become further muted as a form of coping. It is not that children don't feel cold or hungry; rather, these feelings do not become the focus of their perception, and instead their attention becomes habitually directed elsewhere.

In the case of Tūrama School, a uniform policy requires children to wear only prescribed uniform items. Because children often only owned one school sweater or jacket, if this was mislaid, forgotten, or in the wash, many children would come to school underdressed. The uniform policy is not consistently applied—many teachers turn a blind eye to most instances of children wearing nonregulation uniform—however, children will often be admonished or "told off" by senior staff if spotted. This unpredictability of adult sanction means that many children will wear a nonregulation sweater to and from school and in the classroom but remove it to go outside during break times rather than risk punishment. Children could request to borrow an item of "spare uniform," but they tended not to do this out of shyness and fear that they would be embarrassed or questioned.

So, for example, when one chilly morning I sit outside on the deck eating morning snack with Marielle, I am concerned to see her wearing only a T-shirt, with a jacket around her waist. "Aren't you cold?" I exclaim. "Why don't you put your jacket on?" (Figure 6).

Marielle shrugs. "Nah, I'm not cold." She starts talking about something else. But a few minutes later she is huddled against my side, and I see her arms are goose-pimpled. "You are cold! Put on your jacket!"

She shakes her head and mumbles that she'll get in trouble, and I realize the jacket that I mistook for school regulation actually was not.

Children's ability to respond to feeling cold, therefore, is dependent on their ability to conform to the regulations of the institution in which they are placed. The school also constrains children's ability to thermoregulate through other methods; in both of these examples children were placed in situations where they were compelled to sit still—Whetu on a cold gym floor for assembly, Marielle on the steps for lunch-eating time—which prevented their warming themselves through physical activity. The perception of temperature, therefore, is likely developed not only through adult socialization but also in relation to distribution of power and authority, which create constraints on access to the material or bodily resources needed to maintain homeostasis.

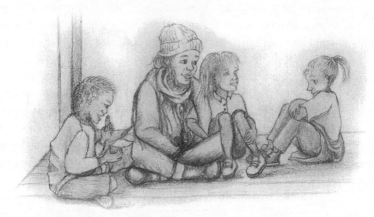

FIGURE 6 "Why don't you put your jacket on?"

Yet, while they were not allowed to warm up, both children in these examples were clearly aware of the cold, as I was—although I was the one drawing Marielle's attention to her goose-pimpled skin, while she did her best to ignore it. Meanwhile others, similarly underdressed, seemed unperturbed.

Such variation in children's cold-sensing abilities is not unexpected, given that children's backgrounds, experiences, and degree of development are far from homogenous. However, it may be important to note that in these examples both Whetu and Marielle had previously been wearing clothing that they were then required to remove. For children who lose clothing, the sharp change in temperature is perhaps felt more keenly than for children who had been underdressed for the whole day. Children who have learned to access what they need to keep them warm have also likely better learned how to read the signals that tell them when more clothing is needed. Unfortunately for children who are powerless to respond to feeling cold, a well-developed sensitivity to cold becomes an impediment to functioning in other areas, directing children's attention toward their ongoing discomfort at the expense of attention to other social or developmental needs. In this context, tuning out cold enables children to focus more attention on socializing and play; the discomfort of cold recedes, though likely still inhibiting full functionality. For a child at Tūrama School, an insensitivity to cold may be an advantage, when there is not anything they could do about it anyway. However, rendering children helpless about feeling cold potentially also disrupts their ability to learn when and how to respond to homeostatic strains on the body—what Freund (1982) describes as "being in touch," or the capacity to monitor and interpret messages of the body and mobilize resources to deal with those messages. Such a disruption of bodily signals and their interpretation can also occur in the regulation of other aspects of the body, including hunger.

The Coproduction of Hunger

This intersection between socialization and material constraints as forces shaping children's bodily perceptions also manifests in experiences of hunger. Bourdieu (1984) uses the notion of "taste" to explain the way in which people develop preferences for what is available to them, where "individuals appropriate as voluntary choices and preferences, lifestyles which are actually rooted in material constraints" (Shilling 1993, 129), and thus the social environment becomes deeply embodied. Bourdieu discusses this manifestation of habitus in terms of classed dietary preferences, stout versus champagne, but here I apply this notion more broadly as a way of understanding the way constraints are given socially constructed meanings and embodied by the children at Tūrama School. Here, a lack of lunch is reframed as "not hungry" and this becomes an embodied "choice," which I argue helps to calibrate the perception of hunger. This modeling of the senses, again, does not occur through traditional socialization but is coproduced out of children's own cultural rules, which are in turn influenced by material constraints.

Research across disciplines suggests that signals such as hunger or satiation are intrinsically biosocial, and the social and cultural milieu may variably interpolate the experience of hunger at the moment of noticing, recognizing, interpreting, or responding to perceptions. In anthropology, Hastrup points out that "while the need for nutrition is universal, the "feeling of hunger" is culturally mediated" (1993, 731); hunger signals can mean different things in different cultures. For example, Scheper-Hughes's (1993) analysis of "*nervoso*" among shantytown dwellers in northeast Brazil demonstrates a collective reinterpreting of chronic hunger as illness in a context in which people had greater ability to obtain medical treatment than sufficient food. An elastic folk illness category ubiquitous across many cultures particularly in the Mediterranean and Latin America, in Brazil a particular medicalized version of nervoso had come to represent the symptoms of collective starvation—wasting, madness, shakiness, irritability, despair—as a personal problem requiring treatment with medication. In this context of chronic food insufficiency and routinized suffering, talk of hunger had become disallowed, fainting or rage represented as a personal deficiency, weakness, or nerves. This reflects a shift in the way the body is perceived in relation to its needs and what those needs imply about the society in which that body resides. While a hungry body needs food, a sick body could be treated with medication, and a prescription for tranquilizers and sleeping pills was obtainable while regular, full meals were not. A hungry body indicates a malfunctioning society, while a sick body is the result of personal misfortune. Meanwhile the impoverished of Brazil came to share the hegemonic medicalized view of themselves through a subtle transformation of everyday knowledge and practices of the body. Being prescribed medication to treat "illness" that is clearly connected to malnutrition reinforced that people and their children were indeed suffering from sickness, a distortion of reality in which the hungry become complicit in reproducing the ideologies and practices that deny what they really need.

In this way, hunger signals may be culturally interpreted or reconstructed as something else, but cultural and social norms can also shape whether or not hunger signals are perceived—or perhaps even produced—in the first place. In psychology, experiments have pointed to a variety of external signals that can cue people to consume food, including sensory cues that are exploited in advertising and culturally normative cues such as portions on plates and structured times of day for eating (Herman and Polivy 2008; Wansink, Painter, and North 2005). For example, Rozin and colleagues (1998) conducted an experiment that found that amnesiac patients who had no recollection of just having consumed a meal would consume a second and then begin a third lunch when the meal was presented to them ten to thirty minutes after the first—despite the fact that their stomachs were physically full. The researchers concluded that the memory of the last culturally defined complete meal was a key factor in mediating bodily cues.

Adult socialization is also a powerful mediator of children's eating. While children are born with the ability to recognize hunger and satiation (Fomon, Filer, Thomas, et al. 1975), adults can often override children's own feelings in ways that can disrupt the ability to self-regulate food intake. A U.S. study of adult communication with children at mealtimes reports a variety of ways that adults cue children to modify their eating, including drawing children's attention to their internal cues—referencing hunger, thirst, or fullness—but also to external cues such as food quantities or the time, encouraging children to eat more or telling children they are done (Ramsay, Branen, Fletcher, et al. 2010). In a seminal experiment, Birch and colleagues (1987) showed that children who are conditioned to notice external cues—for example the amount of food on their plate or rewards for eating—showed less responsiveness to feelings of hunger and satiation than those who were cued to focus on their internal state. The implication is that if the perception of hunger and satiation can be disrupted through social cues, then the relationship among bodily cues, perception, and interpretation must be the outcome of a biosocial coproduction (Lock 2001)—a learned process. And if the production, awareness, or encoding of bodily signals is biosocial in nature, then it follows that when social conditions differ, the way that bodily signals are learned will be different, too, resulting in different embodiments of things like hunger and cold.

Embodying "Not Hungry"

As described in chapter 5, at Tūrama School, every child has the option of requesting a "spare lunch" if they do not come with their own. In theory, the availability of these lunches should mean that every child eats a substantial meal at lunchtime. In reality, the vast majority of children do not. While all children must sit and eat together during the first ten minutes of morning tea and lunchtime—"lunch-eating time"—perhaps a quarter of them will have a sandwich or other substantial food item (such as a pie bought from the local bakery, now cold), about half will be eating only a packet of chips or some cookies, and about a quarter will eat nothing at all.

While it is not unusual for children to not eat lunch in other contexts—teachers at a British school describe a "sandwich graveyard" (Morrison 1996)—variation occurs in the degree to which children's eating habits are seen as "normal" and in the degree of adult intervention. In the school where Morrison conducted her research, parents would be notified about "persistent noneaters" and school rules and supplied lunches were aimed at making sure children had a "proper meal" while supporting parental choice about their child's nutrition. At Tūrama School, the equivalent "proper meal" is the rare exception, while teachers, having limited ability to influence what children eat, are usually more concerned with the proper disposal of rubbish.[4] This difference in what is seen as normal or acceptable by adults as well as children's peer cultures, together with material constraints on what is possible, interact to structure children's eating habits in particular ways. Following Bourdieu, I argue that these habits solidify into routine practices of the body, structuring perceptions and ultimately the health and nutritional status of the body in locally specific ways.

For several weeks at the beginning of fieldwork, at lunchtime I sat next to eleven-year-old Pikau, a physically slight girl who had immediately claimed me as her friend. While I ate my sandwich, Pikau would never eat, instead hunching over her bony knees on the step while she chattered to me about the happenings of the day. Uncomfortable eating beside someone who was not, I would ask her why she wasn't eating, and for weeks she would reply that she wasn't hungry, close off, and change the subject. "Not hungry," I learned, was the standard response I would receive from any child with this question, as predictable as the lack of lunch in the first place.[5] It took me a while to realize that my question was not considered socially appropriate by these children who would happily answer almost anything else. When I stopped asking, Pikau eventually volunteered that she didn't have lunch, explaining, "My mother only makes lunch for my brother, so she can buy me more clothes and toys," which did not clarify things for me.

Yet when children had the opportunity to eat, many of them still did not. I was amused one lunchtime when, after Cassidee told me she wasn't hungry, Dandre gave her a packet of trail mix, which she accepted. Cassidee then proceeded to pick out and eat all of the chocolate chips, and wandered across the field, sprinkling the rest over the grass. It seemed that when she said she wasn't hungry, she was being quite genuine.

Coming from an adult assumption that a child without lunch is a hungry child, and a hungry child wishes to eat, I was perturbed by the chronic undereating and baffled that so few would take up the offer of a free lunch. "Not hungry" was a foreign concept to me when I had grown up on three meals a day and would, after a morning of intense activity, be even more hungry than I would be on a non-school day. As discussed in chapter 4, some of the rejection of spare lunches is likely due to the stigmatized social meaning attached to spare lunches. However, I suggest that the effects of this intersection of material constraints and children's own cultural practices further create a peer socialization and embodiment of "not hungry." Children's embodiment of not hungry is not only about food scarcity but also about how practices of food distribution and consumption are understood as part of a social order and governed by a complicated set of social rules predicated on a sharing economy. In brief, this social order involves an economy of sharing when a resource is plentiful as a strategy for buffering against future uncertainty. While some foods are categorized as "sharing foods," coming with a moral expectation to share, this categorization contrasts with social sanctions shaming against begging for food or "scabbing." As an alternative to scabbing, children may instead use aggressive techniques to intimidate and recategorize food as "sharing food." For those less able to reciprocate in the sharing economy because they rarely or never have lunch, the practice of "not hungry" becomes an alternative to "scabbing," incurring a social debt, or being seen as pōhara, or poor (see chapter 5).

At Tūrama School, as in other places, adults attempt to discourage children from sharing food and drink in order to limit the spread of illness, in particular the streptococcal bacteria that causes strep throat. Many children used the concept of germs to explain the origin of sickness and attributed the cause of specific sickness episodes to the sharing of food or drink. However, sharing is an important aspect of children's sociality and cooperation, as well as a common method of increasing social capital. Bourdieu's (1986) forms of capital, in which accumulated labor takes the form of social or cultural, as well as economic assets, is useful for understanding the micro-economy that underpinned interactions at Tūrama School. While other studies have emphasized the function of ritualized sharing or trade in expressing and regulating children's social relationships (Katriel 1987, 1988; Mishler 1979), the scarcity of resources at Tūrama School means that sharing, steeped in a moral code, also forms the basis of children's economies—an important way of building social capital that can later be translated into the reciprocal use of resources in the future, similar to the strategies Stack (1974) describes as used by black kin and community networks in the U.S. Midwest.

A quotidian example can be seen in the circulation of stationery items such as erasers or sharpeners—a micro-economy I participated in and to some extent took advantage of as a way to compensate for my lack of cultural capital in other areas. Important to note is that such stationery items are both essential and scarce; children need them to complete their work, but they are easily lost, and children have limited ability to replace them. Consequently, children rely on borrowing erasers and such from peers, and to decline is seen as uncooperative or selfish. On the other hand, an eraser is an asset through which the owner can accumulate considerable social capital, building an image of generosity and helpfulness, which can be traded on in future interactions. The more erasers are lent out, however, the quicker they are lost. So when stationery items are incorporated into the sharing economy, ownership of that item—and the opportunity to build social capital—becomes temporary. When I began participating in the classroom, I learned that the best way to engage with and observe children was to join them in their work, and I brought a case of pencils, erasers, sharpeners, and colored pencils for my own use. These items quickly facilitated my entry into the stationery economy—they were admired, borrowed, and inevitably began to disappear—and then I became the one who needed to borrow things. However, since I could much more easily refill my pencil case than my child-peers—even getting reimbursed for my "fieldwork expenses"—I held an advantaged position within this stationery economy, never quite one of them. The principle is that those who have excess resources are expected to share but also gain a lot of credit through sharing, which buffers against the times when resources are scarce.

The sharing of food operates in a similar way, although the rules are complicated by the consumable nature of food; while ten people can use one eraser multiple times, a cookie can be eaten only once. Therefore, children may be expected and pressured to share perceived excess food, especially if the food comes in a form that lends itself easily to sharing, like a large packet of cookies or chips. For example, one day I noticed a trail of children eating wafer sticks, and followed them to find Victor, who was offering a large container to the swarms around him while at the same time protesting, "This is my only lunch!" In this case, it was not the overall quantity of food—the cookies were very light and even a whole tin would not have constituted a substantial lunch for a large boy—but the culturally defined nature of the food. A family-sized container of cookies falls under the category of "sharing food."

On the other hand, the practice of "scabbing" or begging for food from peers is socially unacceptable and stigmatized; annoying for the target, it also represents a shameful public acknowledgement that the child does not have the food they need. To avoid being labeled a "scabber," children may pressure or bully others for a share rather than begging. Performed with a bravado that suggests the demand is reasonable, the more aggressive approach works to redefine the food item in question into the category of "sharing" food, including the moral undertone that comes with it; it would be "stingy" not to share.

Sharing therefore represents a socially acceptable way of redistributing food resources, and social pressure to "not be stingy" can function as a way of prompting children to share. If this strategy does not work, however, children may be accused of "scabbing," which is deeply shameful. One lunchtime, after I produce a sandwich and an apple for my lunch. Kauri, a bigger boy who is friendly but often takes on the role of class bully, leans over to me.

"Oi Miss, what's that?"

"Why are you calling me Miss?"

"I mean Julie. What's that?"

"It's a sandwich."

"Yeah, what kind?"

"Cheese and jam." This causes ripples of surprise among the children nearby.

"Cheese and *jam*?"

"Ew!"

"Nah, it's actually really good," I assure them.

"Oh, can I have it, Miss?" Kauri asks.

"Don't call her Miss, ow!"[6]

I smile but shake my head.

"Oh, please Julie? Please can I have it? Half?" I shake my head again and start eating.

"Can I have your apple, Julie?" Ruby, on my other side asks.

"No, I want it!" Says Ngapaea. "Give it to me."

"You guys have got a whole basket of fruit in your class!" I say. "I saw it before, it's got mandarins and bananas."

"It doesn't have apples," they complain.

Kauri continues, "Oh, can I just have that bit of sandwich?"

"Stop scabbing ow!" I say, and he laughs, amused at my lingo, but withdraws. At this point I start to feel sorry for him, so I call him back, break the sandwich in half, and give it to him.

Then Ngapaea snatches the half left in my hand. "Ew," she says, looking at it.

"Oi! You better eat that now," I say, annoyed. She tastes it and makes a face.

"What is this! I thought it was cheese and mayo."

"It's cheese and jam," I say. "You stole my sandwich and now you're complaining."

"You should have cheese and mayo, and white bread!" she informs me. She stuffs the rest of the sandwich into her mouth, making faces. "This is the worst thing I ever ate," she mumbles through a mouth full of bread.

While I tended to be an easier mark for pressured "sharing," in calling out Kauri's behaviour as "scabbing" I had tapped into a much more powerful social mechanism than I had realized, shaming him in front of his peers. When I called him back, I recast the interaction into the category of "sharing," a shift that was aggressively taken advantage of by Ngapaea, who did not give me a chance to accuse her of scabbing also but stole rather than begged for my food. This episode illustrates that although sharing is socially promoted among children, and pressuring others to share can be an effective way of gaining resources, the tactic also runs the risk of backfiring—especially if used too often—and the child who asks for food may be cast as that most stigmatized being, the scabber.

The difference between children trying their luck, like Kauri, and those who maintain the practice of "not hungry" is, I suggest, in the degree of children's ability to reciprocate in the sharing economy. For many children, lunch is unreliable, and they may have something to eat on some days but not on others. The office lady, in charge of distributing the spare lunches, noticed an increase in demand leading up to the day that weekly government benefits are deposited. Other children were less likely to get lunch towards the end of their parents' pay-week. Children could also forget, lose, or have their lunch stolen. So, for some children, participating in a sharing economy was a strategy to buffer against leaner times. However, for many children, lunches were not just unreliable, but reliably absent. A child who never has lunch may hope for handouts, or scab or bully food from others at the risk of losing social acceptance, but an alternative to asking for food from others is to not need food at all.

By using the phrase "not hungry" I am not suggesting that these children really are not hungry, or that they are not undernourished or not in need of food. Nor am I suggesting that this is "just" their socially accepted discourse. Rather, I suggest this as an example of how the lines between the body and its social performance are not discretely drawn. The "not hungry" body and "not hungry" discourse are not reflections of each other, but mutually constitute each other. In this context, children do not become habituated to eating at lunchtime—or de-habituate themselves (as it is more common for younger children to have lunch that has been prepared by a parent than it is for older children). Instead of risking being seen as scabbers, children may cultivate a bodily practice of "not hungry," which in itself conditions those children to be less tuned in to hunger signals, and may instead focus attention onto other perceptions—a practice that accrues over time into an embodied habitus of "not hungry." In this way, children's cultures create the conditions for their own socialized body.

Who Has a Sore Throat?

My impression of how children were experiencing their bodies in relation to temperature and hunger comes from the disconcerting sense of incongruity with how I was experiencing mine. My analysis of how the rheumatic fever program influences how children are learning to "be" in their bodies is based in part from changes I noticed in the way I related to my body, with the inference that in this case, what I was noticing could parallel how the children habituated to theirs. As I observed teachers asking children about their throats, accompanied children to the clinic, assisted the clinic nurses, and pondered the promotional warnings of the danger of sore throat, I was aware of every scratch and tickle in my own throat. When I came down sick on the last day of term—the cliché of teachers— I spent the holiday convinced that I had strep throat, though without a handy clinic, I never got it checked. It may be a coincidence that during the six-week period in which this chapter was drafted, I twice came down with a cold, the most marked symptom of which was a roaring sore throat. But perhaps not such a coincidence; as I will go on to argue here, there is a vast body of psychological evidence demonstrating a relationship between external cues and subjective symptom experience (Pennebaker 1982).

What I noticed, a "tuning in" to the feeling of the throat, was not a purposeful shaping of children's relationship to their bodies described in much of the child-hood embodiment literature, where parents encouraged or admonished children into a particular way of inhabiting the body. Instead, this internal awareness of the throat came by way of a contingent socialization—the inadvertent and unseen consequence of a repeated cuing toward sore throat by teachers, parents, clinic staff, the media, and other children (detailed in chapter 4). In this way, sore throat becomes highlighted as a significant signal of the body because children's atten-tion is regularly drawn to it: they are asked every day to notice if they have a sore throat, they are affirmed and treated seriously when they self-identify as having a sore throat, and sore throat is linked to anxiety through media portrayals and children's own peer discourse of sore throat. The intervention of the rheumatic fever campaign and throat clinic in this way becomes a new "structuring struc-ture," generating a new form of habitus specific to this generation of children and in this particular nexus of ethnic background and class.

This elevation of sore throat within children's consciousness is reflected in the large numbers flocking to the clinic, a corresponding increase in my own sore throats, and in how often sore throat made an appearance in children's sick-ness discourse. In brainstorms of "kinds of illness," an activity I conducted dur-ing interviews, sore throat was among the most frequently mentioned symptoms, followed closely by rheumatic fever. Unsurprisingly, when I invited children to tell me about a time they remember when they were sick, many stories involved trips to the doctor or school clinic for sore throats. However, sore throats also made appearances in unexpected places. When I interviewed children specifi-cally about their asthma, on a number of occasions children made reference to sore throat. For example, Te Kapua told me the worst thing about asthma is that "it's sore in my throat," and in a follow-up interview several months later, when I asked if he'd had any other symptoms of asthma that month, he said, "I usually play outside but when I—when I had . . . a sore throat, and, um . . . and the asthma came up, I couldn't go outside? So . . . sore throat?"

As a general symptom of childhood illness, mentions of sore throats would not be unexpected among groups of children who did not have a dedicated "sore throat clinic." By comparison however, in another New Zealand study of children's illness experience, this time with four-year-olds, sore throat is mentioned only once (McIntosh 2013). Also notable is that although the Tūrama School clinic also carried out skin checks and treatments—in fact 130 assessments over the period of my fieldwork—this was a much less emphasized aspect of the clinic, and, though they were a common occurrence, children rarely mentioned skin infections. Among countless everyday physical and social ills—colds, eczema, asthma, undernutrition, tiredness—sore throat emerged as culturally salient—unsurprising, given its social highlighting from the adult world, but reinforced through children's shared, visible experiences. That such social highlighting should have an effect on actual perceptions of sore throat is consistent with what a large body of psychological literature would predict.

Psychology of Symptom Perception and Its Cultural Elaboration

The sore-throat clinic intervention—asking children every day if they have a sore throat—emerges from positivist assumptions of a sore throat as an objective symptom, like bleeding or fever: if a child has a sore throat, they will already be aware of it, and if the child doesn't have a sore throat, they will know. Of course, like hunger and cold and other forms of pain, sore throat is a subjective symptom, and—if children share the adult understanding of the term in the first place—one that is produced out of a complicated set of socio-psycho-biological processes. Given the vast psychological literature documenting the relationship between external cues and subjective symptoms (Pennebaker 1982, 2000), it seems likely that children's experience of sore throat at Tūrama School represents field evidence of at least some phenomena that reliably occur in experimental settings.

Of particular relevance is research that demonstrates how attention to a given sensation can alter how people can perceive sensory stimulation. In a classic series of studies, Pennebaker and colleagues investigated the effects of "priming" on symptom perception; participants who were primed to expect or notice symptoms did indeed report the symptoms as expected, compared with control groups (Pennebaker 1982). This "priming" may be seen as analogous to the prompting of children to notice sore throats at Tūrama School. In one experiment, after filling out a checklist of common physical symptoms, Pennebaker's participants were asked to close their eyes and concentrate according to the one of four attention conditions: noticing nasal congestion (congestion increase), free breathing through the nose (congestion decrease), sensations that occurred while breathing through the nose (congestion neutral), and a non-bodily distraction (N=48). After a second questionnaire, it was found that groups' perceptions of congestion changed significantly according to how they had been directed to attend—those who were asked to notice congestion reported increases in congestion; those who were directed to notice free breathing reported decreased congestion—while subjects in the neutral and distraction conditions changed very little. The effect was so great that three participants—all in the congestion increase group—blew their noses directly after the experiment, while a participant from the decrease group reported her nose had never felt so clear in weeks and suspected the room had been sprayed with a decongestant. It can be imagined how a similar effect may occur when children are asked every day to notice whether they have a sore throat.

Such evidence of psychological mediators in symptom perception offers insight into the way in which a shared cultural environment could shape the perceptory experiences of a collective group of people through psychological mechanisms, creating local variations in sensory modes. Such psychological mechanisms are likely not universal, but also shaped by local cultural meanings and values that influence the interpretation of bodily sensations—for example, translating symptoms into culturally recognized categories of "sickness" (Young 1982). As detailed in chapter 4, Christensen (1999) demonstrates that as children learn to interpret and classify their subjective experience of the body, they come to understand, first, that some bodily sensations of discomfort or pain are accepted as "normal" and others are not and, second, that some sensations indicate the need for intervention or treatment and others are acceptable. In this case, children at Tūrama School are learning that the symptoms termed "sore throat" are important and threatening, while for children in other areas of the country—white, more affluent children—sore throat appears to be a much less salient aspect of this classification process.

I want to emphasize, however, that an important part of the process is learning not only to interpret and classify bodily sensations but also to learn—or unlearn—to notice and feel signals like hunger, cold, and sore throat in the first place. As Husserl describes intentionality, amid a sea of sensory inputs, perception faces "toward" some as others recede (cf. Desjarlais and Throop 2011, 90), including perceptions from within the body. As one feeling among a body-full of various discomforts, pains, and even pleasures, the internal state of the throat is not something that children are necessarily conscious of. Even children suffering from severe cases of strep throat, with swollen "soccer balls" for tonsils, would often be picked up in class checks because they hadn't come forward for treatment. Perhaps, Whaea Allison thought, this was out of fear or wariness, or because they just hadn't realized this symptom wasn't normal, or because they did not know that *this* is what was meant by "sore throat." It seemed, however, that sometimes children were simply not aware of any soreness. Like the "not hungry" and "not cold" children, for these children, sore throat was not something they had learned to recognize, or possibly even to notice.

On the other hand, once children have learned to notice a bodily signal, they may become *particularly* tuned into that sensation, and this may help to explain the large number of children coming to the clinic. The regular discursive "highlighting" of sore throat, the routinized surveillance from clinic staff and from children themselves as their teacher daily draws their attention to the feeling of their throat, and the imbuing of sore throat with anxiety and threats of death, brings a parallel "tuning in" and heightened awareness—a "highlighting"—of the feeling of one's throat. For most children who presented regularly, coming to the clinic appeared to be a positive experience of receiving adult care and attention. Such positive reinforcement made it more likely that children who experienced a sore throat would come to be checked again; however, it also works in tandem with the provocative promotional campaign to motivate children's awareness of their throats and the sensitized perception of any small discomforts. As children became more aware of sore throat, they become more sensitized to the subtle variations of sensations of the throat, picking up the tickle of "eating scratchy food," the dryness of thirst, and the tenderness from "talking too much." Without understanding the etiology of strep throat, all of these are classified as the same, threatening "sore throat" and verified as such through the clinic processes—a self-referential feedback loop that reinforces the prevalence of this risk. Moreover, children who do become habituated toward sore throat are more likely to get their strep throat picked up and treated, meaning that variation in habitus becomes magnified by corresponding variation in health care. This marks the beginning of biosocial differentiation that can end in unequal bodies.

Conclusion

This particular confluence of resource limitations, cultural norms, and social interventions collectively lay out the structure for a form of habitus where the state of the throat emerges in prominence, while other bodily sensations such as hunger and temperature recede. Although there is variation—not all children experience their body in this way—I suggest the presence of a trend toward this particular configuration, also depending on personal circumstances that shape children's access to resources.

This represents a way of "being" in the body that is not only culturally distinct but also particular to this subgroup of children at this time and place. Children may develop perceptions of their bodies that may be distinct from adults in the community, shaped by "structuring structures" that vary from the environments of adults, and including structures that children themselves generate. At a structural level, constraints on children's ability to respond to perceptions of cold or hunger may work to mute those perceptions, as children "tune out" discomfort that they are powerless to alleviate, and "tune in" to other stimuli such as social interactions. Meanwhile, children's peer cultures comprise complex social norms and rules that shape how children may express or respond to perceptions, potentially influencing the experience of those perceptions.

Finally, social interventions—in this case, because of new health policy—may inadvertently create new structures that condition children to experience their bodies in a particular way, enhanced by the social meanings children create around these interventions for themselves. In these ways, children can be seen as coproducing the conditions for their own embodiment. While children's perceptions of bodily signals may, as they grow up, eventually converge with those of their parents, there is potential for childhood tuning into sore throat or out of hunger to set in place trajectories of bodily practices that are carried into adulthood, with particular implications for health. Turning the lens of analysis close to the body can therefore reveal how deep the biosocial dialectic—and the foundations of the social production of health—play out.

7

Practicing Resilience

At ten years old, Cassidee was close to the shortest in the class, but held herself with a kind of calm poise that always gave me the sense that I was already looking at her adult self, just in miniature. She had mastered the cool tilt of the chin and raised eyebrow that adults would use to greet one's "bros," and while friendly enough, she had an insularity that suggested you could talk to her or not—she would be content either way.

Cassidee had been through five changes of school in as many years, and when I interviewed her in term three she commented—as if it were of little consequence—that her aunt intended for the family to move again at the end of the year. It was common for children who were new to the school to associate more with me. I was a secure base to work from as they tackled the task of negotiating foreign social networks and finding their place in the system. At the start of the year, Cassidee, new to the school and half the size of some children, hovered at the outskirts of the group of girls at lunch-eating time and was the lone girl in her class to go swimming in the pool at playtime. After the pool closed for the winter she would line up for her turn on the spinners, which did not require a social group to play on. When she wasn't on the playground I might find her wandering alone or with another straggler, and she would come to me for a hug and a chat. When I spent the day in her class, she would sit next to me on the mat. Whenever she saw me—whether for the first time that day or the tenth—she would greet me in a sing-song "HI, Jool-*lay*," to which I would reply with a matching "HI, Cassi-*day*," and she would smile.

Within a couple of months I spotted Cassidee walking along with another girl, Gemma, with swapped shoes so they were both wearing one of each. I commented on this to the boy I was standing with, Caleb, and he confirmed "that means they're BFFs [best friends forever]". This symbolic advertisement of friendship tended to occur when connections were newly forming. However, while a tentative bond might have been forged, Cassidee retained her independence, casually joining in games but less frequently engaging in the physical closeness characteristic of intimate friendships.

Cassidee's father had died, and she usually lived with her mother, who at forty-five was considered by the children to be particularly old, and thirteen-year-old brother, although Cassidee has many other siblings she does not know. As noted in chapter two, whānau are often fluid and shifting, and at the time I interviewed her, Cassidee was living with an aunt while her mother had moved in with an elder daughter to help take care of a new baby.

Cassidee's story is not that of a typical New Zealand child, but it does include many of the features of a childhood life that are distinctly more common among the children at Tūrama School than in other areas of the country—the consequence of generations of structural disadvantage, as described in chapter 2. These features—transience, shifting family circumstances, and loss—create a life that is lived on the edge of certainty, not only for these children who are directly affected by instability and grief, but also for those around them who bear witness to and imagine as their own the experiences of their classmates. Produced through a social ecology shaped by economic, political, and cultural forces, this vulnerability is not passively experienced by children like Cassidee, but actively responded to through practices that may become culturally normative ways of being among their peers. These practices, I argue, form the basis of resilience, the processes through which children, with agency, employ strategies in response to perceptions of vulnerability to navigate their circumstances.

As a reframing of risk that focuses on how individuals overcome adversity to thrive, the concept of resilience has proved remarkably popular over the past four decades. Yet exactly what resilience is and how it can be identified, measured, and fostered are still subjects of wide debate (Barber 2013; Bonanno and Diminich 2013; Masten 2001; Rutter 2013). In particular, one question has been the role of children's coping in models of resilience. This question recognizes the tension between structure and agency that is central to the coproduction of health, but also reflects a second tension between competing constructions of children as vulnerable and in need of protection on the one hand, and as having agency and competence on the other (Ungar 2012). Recently, researchers (Ungar, Brown, Liebenberg, et al. 2008; Ungar 2011; Ungar 2012) have proposed a socio-ecological framework to help to resolve the former tension, and such a framework, I would suggest, also serves to reconcile the latter.

While traditional child-centric approaches to resilience have tended to place responsibility on children for coping, approaches that neglect to incorporate children's experience and activities into the analysis can erase children's agency or run the risk of environmental determinism. In a socio-ecological view, resilience is produced through *interactions* between children and their environment, recognizing the constraints and opportunities produced by specific environments while also making room for what children perceive, experience, and do as significant aspects of those interactions (Ungar 2011). This approach also supports the use of culturally specific lenses for understanding local norms of risk and well-being, including the way that children's views may differ from those of adults.

Such a framework for resilience has been successfully applied in some large-scale research (Eggerman and Panter-Brick 2010; Panter-Brick, Eggerman, Gonzalez, et al. 2009, 2011; Panter-Brick and Eggerman 2012), but not as yet to many ethnographic studies of children. In this chapter I use a socio-ecological framework to unpack dimensions of children's vulnerability and resilience: how the local environment contributes to children's experiences of vulnerability, and how they respond to those experiences through creative practices. The ethnographic focus here—on a group of children, over time, in the site where they spend a large proportion of each day—allows insight into characteristics of resilience processes that are less visible in the large-scale quantitative studies more typical of resilience research. While being mindful of Ungar's (2011) call to decentralize the child from resilience research in favour of ecologies, I aim to show that an understanding of children's ecologies is incomplete without including children's activities and perspectives, because, as with their health, children are active in the coproduction of their environment, and their experiences shape the way they negotiate their circumstances toward their own care practices. At the same time, the socio-ecological resilience concept helps to reveal new dimensions of children's practices: as interconnected with other individuals; as sometimes unrecognized forms of resilience; and as accommodations, with buffering in one domain coming at a cost in another.

These features of resilience practices may be briefly illustrated in Cassidee's story. While some children cling to social connections for the protections they can offer, Cassidee's experience is that school connections are temporary, and so she has come to mainly rely on herself. The strategies children use to cope with their vulnerability are not limitless, however, but closely bound to the specific ecological contexts that children both inhabit and help to coproduce. These contexts constrain and shape children's social power, resources, and possible strategies, while their practices in turn coproduce their social ecology, often creating new vulnerabilities in the process. Cassidee found a resource in the form of the unthreatening anthropologist hanging out in her classroom. But time spent with an adult means less time spent with peers, and it was only later in the year, when I was spending more time in other classrooms, that she began to form tentative friendships with others. Thus, practices of resilience are often accommodations; they come at a cost, whether because the practices are associated with new forms of risk, or because a practice that is successful in one domain creates a disadvantage in another, or because a practice that benefits one child makes another more vulnerable.

Thus, by tracing the specific strategies that children at Tūrama School employ, it becomes clear that the vulnerabilities and practices of individual children are inextricably linked to those of the people around them. As children operate within their social ecology, they simultaneously coproduce the conditions that open up or constrain vulnerabilities and resources for themselves and their peers. This is not to say that children are responsible for their environment— the circumstances children face at Tūrama School are largely a result of social, political, and economic processes that are beyond the control of their parents, let alone the children themselves. But it is to suggest that individuals cannot be viewed independently of the others with whom they interact, because their vulnerabilities and practices are interconnected.[1]

Practices, here, are also borne through the body, which plays a dominant role in children's experience and functions as a tool in practices of resilience. A second thread of my analysis therefore spotlights the body within resilience practices as an important locus through which these processes can be traced. Children's biological immaturity renders them twice vulnerable; they are physically less powerful, but also their immaturity is often used to justify further constraint of their power and agency in the name of "protection."[2] The body is a medium through which feelings of vulnerability can be expressed but is also a key resource for children's practices of resilience: through self-care practices of the body; through using their physical competence to threaten or defend; or through using their vulnerable appearance to elicit care. These embodied practices of resilience contribute to local, often gendered norms within children's subcultures and create new vulnerabilities for children who find themselves at the receiving end of exclusion, aggression, or violence. This focus on what children do, and how vulnerability and resilience are expressed through practices of the body, also allows for an analysis of the accommodations made for resilience.

The Resilience Paradigm and Socio-ecological Frameworks

In psychology, resilience frameworks seek to avoid a deficit model of the relationship between adverse circumstances and poor outcomes by instead focusing on the protective factors that help young people to mitigate risk and achieve success (Luthar and Cicchetti 2000; Masten 2001; Rutter 1987). Risk, in this context, refers to variables that increase the likelihood of immediate or later psychopathy or "negative outcomes" (Goyos 1997, as cited in Boyden and Mann 2005). Despite the optimism of the approach, resilience remains a nebulous concept, variably defined,[3] and with great debate over whether it constitutes a trait, a process, or an outcome; how useful it is; what it is really measuring; and the problems of operational definitions of risk, protective factors, and positive and negative "outcomes."

Traditionally, resilience research has oriented toward quantitative, longitudinal studies, with the aim of identifying the predictors of well-being (variably defined) following adversity (Bonanno and Diminich 2013). This research does not usually attend to children's perceptions and experiences but instead relies on normative (i.e., adult) assessments of what constitutes risk, adversity, and outcomes, and tends to generalize broad patterns at a population level. So, resilience may be measured through "outcomes" such as "pro-sociality," physical growth, or school attendance, while "symptoms" or other manifestations of trauma or distress suggest a "lack" of resilience. This research has contributed significant understanding of what influences children's well-being—in particular, the importance of at least one supportive relationship with an adult (Boyden and Mann 2005). Increasingly, however, the normative operationalizing of the resilience concept has been problematized, for example through questions about the generalizability of protective factors across cultures. Likewise, the designation of variables as risks, negative outcomes, or signs of resilience has been shown to reflect normative assumptions of the causes and effects of distress. Contrary to what might be expected, for example, Panter-Brick and Eggerman (2012) find that among their Afghan participants, family conflict, rather than political violence, is the most salient cause of distress. Other scholars have argued that individuals can be resilient and also show symptoms of post-traumatic stress disorder (PTSD) (Yehuda and Flory 2007), and that dropping out of school may be an adaptive social strategy for marginalized young people (Dei 1997). This has led to greater attention to context, with an emphasis on defining "outcomes" according to local cultural concepts of, for example, "the good enough life" (Panter-Brick and Leckman 2013) or "doing well" (Ungar, Brown, Liebenberg, et al. 2007).

The emphasis on normative values and perceptions of risk is useful for understanding emic views of resilience but can shift focus from what children do to cope with adversity. This shift is in part a result of an ongoing tension between agency and structure in resilience research. Early trait- and coping-based research was critiqued for tasking the individual with the locus of control, essentially holding children responsible for their own survival (Ungar 2012). Similar critiques have been made from indigenous perspectives; for example, Penehira and colleagues (2014) show how states have co-opted the language of resilience as a neoliberal tool to shift responsibility for survival onto Māori and other indigenous peoples, rather than addressing the contemporary injustices and historical trauma these peoples are required to survive. Meanwhile, models of resilience that focus on "protective factors" in environments can tend to position children and young people in a passive role; they develop resilience because of what adults do, either by providing the conditions to facilitate development and inner strength or by fostering strong social relationships with the child. Shifting the locus of control from the child onto the social and physical environment reinforces the invisibilizing of children's experience and agency, rendering their perceptions, responses, and strategies as by-products of adult interventions.

The socio-ecological approach goes some way toward resolving this tension. Based on Bronfenbrenner's (1979) bio-social-ecological systems model of human development, the model—developed most comprehensively by Michael Ungar—conceptualizes children as placed within ecologies, navigating risk and negotiating resources according to the possibilities available to them (Ungar, Brown, Liebenberg, et al. 2008; Ungar 2011; Ungar 2012). Resilience, therefore, becomes the process of "harnessing" (Panter-Brick and Leckman 2013) or "navigating and negotiating" resources in culturally specific ways (Ungar 2011). This way of thinking about resilience includes children's agency, while recognizing that their resourcefulness is constrained and shaped by the specifics of their local ecological context.

Recent research has applied this framework in large-scale, culturally specific studies of resilience (Eggerman and Panter-Brick 2010; Panter-Brick and Eggerman 2012; Ungar, Brown, Liebenberg, et al. 2007, 2008). In particular, Ungar led an international mixed-methods comparative study of eighty-nine young people aged twelve to twenty-three across eleven countries identified as "doing well" in the face of risk according to local norms (Ungar, Brown, Liebenberg, et al. 2007). For example, fourteen-year-old Saleem painted a relatively positive picture of his life in a Palestinian refugee camp, describing a close-knit peer network who connected him to a collective cause, feelings of self-efficacy, and access to political power, all of which enhanced his sense of identity and cultural adherence. He described small collective acts of resistance—for example, throwing stones at the Israeli army—that contributed to his sense of power and control, and attending school as a way to contribute to the future of a Palestinian state. It is the specific social and political circumstances that create the pathways for Saleem to find a sense of well-being in this way, while young people in other contexts will have qualitatively different patterns in their approach to the social injustices, danger, and relationships they experience. In this research, therefore, resilience is envisaged as dynamic processes that are mediated by young people's culture, context, and resources. This represents a shift from earlier resilience research, in which "shopping lists" of risk and protective factors are employed to discriminate between "resilient" and "non-resilient" individuals, who are dislocated from any socio-economic or cultural context (Layne, Warren, Watson, et al. 2007).

This reframing of resilience invites more detailed ethnographic work to examine the particularities of how children experience vulnerability and negotiate risk and resources toward resilience: the ways contexts open up or constrain pathways, and the way these strategies may set children on particular health trajectories. Usefully, within this ecological framework, it is possible to think of children as practitioners in their own health care, recognizing their agency and efficacy without putting responsibility on them for coping. Children's practices here include negotiation of resources, as well as the interpretive process of recognizing risk, expressing vulnerability, and employing tactics and strategies (de Certeau 1988). An ethnographic understanding of these practices in context is important because children's vulnerability and resilience are, first, shaped by their subjective experience, and second, not produced independently of the vulnerabilities and resilience practices of those with whom children share their social worlds. Indeed, as this chapter will show, the ways that children experience vulnerability are influenced by the social ecologies they themselves collectively coproduce—ecologies that also enable and constrain their practices of resilience. Finally, children's practices, while mitigating some vulnerabilities, may be seen as accommodations in that they create new forms of vulnerability for children or their peers. It is thus useful not only to look at children's resilience in the context of events, experiences, and cultural values, but also within networks of individuals who are all actively negotiating vulnerability and resilience.

Feeling Vulnerable

The majority of resilience research has not accounted for children's emic perspectives of their own vulnerability and coping. Yet if resilience is conceptualized as a set of interactions or practices, then how children perceive their environment and experience their vulnerability will shape the form that these practices take. Contrary to its appropriation as an index of risk in models of children's social and health outcomes, vulnerability is a subjective feeling, the experience of which does not necessary co-vary with statistical or epidemiological models of risk. Nichter (2003, 14) describes vulnerability as referring to the actual feeling of susceptibility to illness or misfortune: a state of weakness, fear, or worry. In this sense, children are made vulnerable, but they also can *feel* vulnerable, an experience that may be related to their socially produced powerlessness but could vary considerably from adult assumptions of what makes children vulnerable (Boyden and Mann 2005; Christensen 2000). What greatly challenges children—such as navigating shifting school peer networks—does not necessarily match adult perceptions of children's vulnerabilities. Meanwhile the concerns of adults about children—such as lower academic achievement caused by transience—do not necessarily form part of children's experience of vulnerability. Because children use perceptions of vulnerability to guide their practices, an understanding of what makes children feel vulnerable and how they respond to these feelings must underpin any understanding of children's resilience.

Yet children's perceptions of risk or feelings of vulnerability rarely appear on the radar in health policy, which assumes that children are passive recipients of care. For example, at Tūrama School, children have a perception that the risk of rheumatic fever is much higher than the epidemiological risk. This perception comes from interpretations of their experience; as described in chapter 4, more than half of the children have been given antibiotics for strep throat at some point since the clinic opened, and from this fact many infer that they either already have or are a step away from having rheumatic fever. Children observe others getting antibiotics and see susceptibility as common; for some children, just the nurse swabbing them is an indication that they are at risk. Combined with the media message that rheumatic fever can cause death, this creates a perception of a much higher risk than the epidemiological data would suggest: "I didn't want to die. 'Cause on the ad, him! He almost died!" Amberlee, age ten, tells me. While in a given population with high exposure to GAS strains only 3–6 percent of individuals will develop rheumatic fever (Carapetis, Currie, and Mathews 2000), the children getting swabbed are unaware that they are most likely not even susceptible. Furthermore, it is rare for a child to die of rheumatic fever; most rheumatic fever-related deaths are in adulthood from the complications of rheumatic heart disease (Wilson 2010). The proximity of death suggested by the media campaign contributes to a perception not only that rheumatic fever is common and easy to contract, but that the consequences are more severe than is the clinical prognosis.

Children's frequent use of the clinic therefore becomes much more understandable when viewed in terms of their own sense of vulnerability. The clinic represents a powerful, accessible resource in mitigating risk through its promise to detect and treat the sore throats that lead to rheumatic fever. The clinic also works with children's agency; in most cases children decide when they need to go to the clinic and put their names forward, children are free to see the nurse during break times, and together with their parents children may take an active role in managing their antibiotics. The fact that children are not helpless in the face of their perceived risk may work to reduce their sense of vulnerability, and the clinic thus gets co-opted into a practice of resilience.

Understanding this relationship between children's experiences, perceptions, agency, and resources is important for understanding not only children's health care practices, but also the impact of a health intervention such as the clinic. As adults have inadvertently created conditions in which children perceive they are at risk of rheumatic fever, adults have also rendered children—and their parents—dependent on the clinic to mitigate their sense of vulnerability. When I asked one of the children's mothers, Anna, how it would be if the clinic closed, she visibly panicked:

> What could I do as a mum, stand and scream. I would stand wherever—the Beehive [Parliament], if I could afford—I would go up there and I would tell them what for. I would rather have my son come in once a week or,

you know, however many times in a week to prevent him getting it, than have him get it because we don't have it so local and so close. . . . Like me and his dad would definitely lose our jobs because there is no way I am having a sick child in hospital and not being with him. And the stress alone would be too much so I reckon we would both lose our jobs, we would have no money to live on. . . . Don't tell me they're shutting it down.

Having had her son Anton come back positive for strep twice, the threat of rheumatic fever is a frightening reality that Anna takes very seriously. For her, the clinic in the school has come to represent the linchpin holding together a family struggling on the edge of coping. Probably in part because of Anna's encouragement, Anton was one of the children who presented at the clinic every couple of weeks to be checked. So long as the clinic remained in the school, it gave the family an accessible resource for managing their vulnerability and, in doing so, practicing resilience. Hence, attention to what makes children and families feel vulnerable in specific contexts is essential for understanding how they "negotiate resources" toward resilience.

Vulnerability and Resilience in Social Networks

In the context of Tūrama School, a significant part of children's experience of vulnerability is produced against a backdrop of a shifting, unpredictable social landscape, where connections are temporary and peer networks are continuously reconfigured. This local ecology is a result of wider structural factors, including the legacy of colonization, a housing crisis, and demographic changes, but is also co-constructed by the children themselves, who actively respond to their vulnerabilities through creating and strategically navigating their peer cultures (Corsaro 1992; Spray, Floyd, Littleton, et al. 2018). Thus, children's vulnerabilities are produced through the interaction of structural forces and children's own interpretive meaning-making, while their responses can create new forms of vulnerability for themselves and others.

I focus here on children's peer ecology at school, as this is where I was based, but the processes—or characteristics of processes—that emerge are likely to be relevant in other domains as well. I follow a growing body of research documenting children's peer groups as important sources of social support (Boyden, Eyber, Feeny, et al. 2004; Boyden and Mann 2005; Spray et al. 2018), although with the caveats that these social practices may not look like the adult view of what is best for children and that practices that are protective for one child can be detrimental to another. The significance of peer networks as a cause of distress for children has tended to be overlooked in resilience research in favor of forms of vulnerability that are more visible to adults: domestic conflict, political violence, environmental catastrophe (but see Boyden et al. [2004] for children's perceptions of peer abuse as the worst consequence of poverty). In this analysis, I aim to bring to light the complexity of children's practices within the peer ecology children themselves coproduce.

As is reflected in Cassidee's story, a high rate of transience is a notable feature of school life, and classes experienced a change in membership of up to 25 percent over the course of the year. Aside from the impact of transience on educational achievement—a factor the teachers would lament—this revolving door of children created a constantly shifting dynamic in classes. The onus was on the new students to integrate themselves, and for many this was a long, slow process. Cassidee, experienced as she was at transitions, took this in her stride, and self-sufficiency seemed to be her strategy for adaptation. She didn't reject friendships, but she didn't actively invest in them to the degree of some of her peers. Other new children sought to build intimacies with a kind of urgency, and in the absence of success elsewhere, girls in particular would cling to me, claiming their spot on the mat next to me and pressing their thighs snug against mine. As the weeks went on and their own connections grew, they would gradually leave me behind and find their own place in the social order.

It was hard for those who arrived, and likewise hard for those who left. Sometimes children had a month or two of notice before the move and would talk about it, naming that they were leaving to friends, teachers, and myself. Children did not tend to talk about how they felt or what the move might mean, but the naming to others, over and over again, put words to the significance of the event and their disturbance. The children hearing in turn would "tell others," who would go back to the leaving child for confirmation and ask, "Are you leaving?" This "naming" would continue up until the child left. Children would also identify whether the child would or would not be present for upcoming events, mapping out the future landscape. When practicing for a choir performance, one girl made it clear to those around her that she would have left before the event took place.

When notice had been given that a child was leaving, a class would sometimes acknowledge or celebrate their last day. Often, however, children would suddenly disappear. Sometimes there had been a few days' notice; sometimes children would simply not return after the holidays. Sometimes children would know they were likely leaving but not know for sure or not know when. My first encounter with this phenomenon is when Ben, a friendly boy who often hangs around me at play times, tells me that he "thinks" this might be his last day. "Oh really?!" I say in surprise, and comment that he'll miss being in the school play, which he has a main role in.

"Yeah," Ben replies. "I think I have to go live with my auntie."

"You think you have to go?"

"Yeah. My social worker? She said I have to go and live with my auntie."

"Oh, wow," I respond. "How do you feel about that?"

Ben shrugs. "I wonder what school I will go to?"

"Do you like your auntie?" I ask.

Ben smiles, "Yeah."

Ben indeed did not come back to school the next day, and if I hadn't happened to stop and chat to him while he hung off the rail outside his classroom, he would have been another unflagged disappearance. As a lead role in the school play, Ben's leaving was of most inconvenience to the teacher directing, who had to hastily replace him. For me, Ben was the first child with whom I had built a relationship who disappeared in this way, and I was shocked at the suddenness of his announcement and the uncertainty he expressed in this final conversation; he didn't know for sure he was going or when, or what his new life would look like, or what school he would be attending the next day.

Moving was hard for those who left but also could be hard for those who were left behind. Friendship bonds could be abruptly broken, leaving children unexpectedly vulnerable and without their closest ally. Ruby, whom we met in chapter 2, had been friends with Eponi since the previous year when, as year fives in a mostly year-six class and on the edge of social circles, they had paired up. This year, Ruby had found herself in a new class with Eponi, the only classmate who had transitioned with her, solidifying her bond. In an interview, Ruby, supported by her new friends Ngapaea and Alexandra, describes the loss of Eponi several months prior:

"It's hard for me "cause my best friend left. And I never got to say goodbye because I had to go to my cousin's *tangi* [funeral] . . ." she trails off. "Eponi, she moved to Wellington I think."

"Because of her dad," Alexandra supplies.

Ruby corrects, "No, "cause of her—"

"Grandpa?" fills in Ngapaea. The three of them tend to build stories in a sort of collaborative project.

"And so, did you know she was leaving?" I wonder.

"Yeah, she told us, she had to go—"

"—to a tangi."

"So how far in advance did you know that Eponi was leaving?"

Ruby hesitates. "Um . . . I don't know."

I clarify, "I mean, was it like she told you one day and the next day she was leaving, or . . . ?"

"No, she told me one day, and then like—oh, she stayed for a week. And then on Friday she left, and that's when I went away," Ruby explains.

This shifting social landscape leaves children with low social capital and few strong social connections in a vulnerable position. Secure acceptance into a bigger group therefore is enormously beneficial. When I interview Ruby later in the year, she is now a core member of a tight, exclusive group of five girls. Ruby and her two friends describe how their group has explicit rules and roles and wields threat of exclusion to keep membership and behavior in line. They had kicked another girl, Soraya, out of the group because of the behavior of her brother. Likewise, they threatened to exclude another girl, Sarah, when she broke the rules and continued to talk to Soraya.

"So you guys feel safe in your group?" I ask.

"Now," Ruby explains, "now—'cause we got a leader."

"Her," Alexandra and Ngapaea both point to Ruby.

"And a co-captain . . ." Ruby adds.

"Me," says Alexandra. "Oh, no—"

"You're the choreographer," Ngapaea corrects.

"You guys are quite structured now," I note.

Ruby agrees. "Yeah because like our—like we're tryna keep it together but—I've been bossing them around, so I have to stop that."

"Yeah but, um, [Sarah] kept on talking to Soraya and telling her what we've been like saying, and talking about—"

"'Cause we got rules," says Ruby.

"Yeah, we got rules. Don't hang out with the haters. Like, haters don't hang out with the haters."

"And no putting your hair on the side."

In the face of forces out of her control that took away her friend, Ruby here has done what is in her power: seized leadership of a group (instead of one close friend) and created a kind of group culture that promotes the loyalty of those friends, ensuring a more stable social positioning and buffer against future losses.

Though Ruby might be described as resilient, it is perhaps more useful to note the forms that her practices of resilience take within this context, how she has come to arrive at her current strategy, and the effect of these practices for her and for others. Her practices both are produced out of her specific experiences of vulnerability but also, at the same time, render others (Soraya and Sarah) more vulnerable. In this way vulnerability and resilience are mutually constituting; vulnerability is produced through the interaction of social conditions and the actions of individuals with agency, while resilience is enacted through agentive practices within the constraints of those same social conditions. A socioecological model recognizes such ecologies as dynamic and shifting networks that are coproduced by the children while they simultaneously jockey to navigate their resources in response to perceptions of vulnerability.

Embodied Vulnerability and Resilience

Although children hugged me, and cried to me, and interrogated me, and showed off their skills on the playground, the times when they came to silently stand next to me marked a different kind of need. They might lean against me, or sit with their thigh pressed against mine, but they said nothing, and if I asked questions or commented it felt like I was speaking the wrong language. They would stay by me for a minute or two and then move on, ready to enter their world again. These were the moments for the things that could not be expressed in words. This, I came to realize, was the language of vulnerability.

Stepping away from ethnocentric definitions and capturing the local cultural norms of risk and resilience invite a particular attention to language; the vocabulary, values, and stories that participants use to construct and express the meaning of experiences. This "meaning-making" has been discussed as core to promoting resilience within constructivist or cultural resilience research (Theron and Theron 2011), which identifies concepts or values expressed in local narratives and ties these to a determination to survive or overcome adversity. For example, Eggerman and Panter-Brick describe adherence to six cultural values as forming the basis of resilience in Afghanistan (2010), while the concept of "sumud—a determination to exist through being steadfast and rooted to the land" was drawn out of analysis of narratives from Palestinian young people (Nguyen-Gillham, Giacaman, Naser, et al. 2008), and in South Africa a cooperative philosophy called "Ubuntu" or "Botho" underpins making sense of poverty (Theron and Theron 2011). These concepts, distilled from interviews with adolescents, young adults, or caregivers, codify vulnerability and resilience into language in a way that I struggled to replicate in my observations of the children of Tūrama School—not because children do not make meaning, but because they did not tend to articulate this meaning verbally. Instead, the experiences of younger people may be better read through embodied expressions of vulnerability and resilience: what they do, how they use their bodies, micro-interactions in the context of their local environments. Such embodied expressions are not unique to children, of course, but have been noted by other authors as particularly relevant to phenomenological studies of children. For instance, Das (1989) notes that children traumatized by anti-Sikh riots in Delhi would not offer extended verbal accounts of their feelings, but knowledge and memories were encoded in their bodies and expressed through displaying injuries, miming events, and projecting the dead into ghosts whose voices haunted them at night. Memories and meaning-making were not bounded within each individual child but held and signified collectively; for children who did not speak, other children spoke for them, naming the spot where a parent had died in a way that mirrors the naming of a loss by the children at Tūrama School. Such interconnected expressions of vulnerability could be similarly traced through the embodied practices of Tūrama School children. The stories in this chapter illustrate vulnerabilities that are expressed through silence and touch, and resilience practiced through bodily power, agency, and autonomy, through the embodiment of sore throat and its vigilant care, the language of aggression, or the shared language of pain.

Mila

At age ten Mila had a quiet maturity that both made her an attractive friend to the girls in her class and endeared her to the teaching staff. Bright and watchful, she would get on with her work while the other children squabbled over stolen erasers and exchanged notes. When I wandered around the school, or stood observing, I would often turn to find her standing next to me, watching too.

Mila lives in a two-bedroom house in, according to her, "quite a bad neighborhood." At the time I interview her, she lives with her mother and an adult cousin, and shares her bedroom with three of her brothers, aged between sixteen and four.

Mila loves her father. He has her name tattooed on his back because she's his favorite daughter, his "good girl," because, Mila tells me, "I listen. I . . . concentrate. I do my chores. I never . . . I never run away from him—well, one time . . . Just one time. And I respect him." Mila tells me she feels safe when he's around. He loves her.

Mila explains that her mother is "almost dying," sick with something the family don't really understand but which the doctor says can't be cured. "And," Mila tells me in her interview, "she's always got a sore shoulder, also neck, because of my dad. Yeah, he, when he was younger, he used to be a Black Power."

I wonder how her father's gang affiliations had impacted her mother's shoulder and neck. Mila explains to me:

"Well, there was this one, there was this one day, and there was this one day, um, my mum and my dad were sleeping next to each other, and then my dad got up and he was all angry, 'cause he wasn't supposed to stay there, 'cause he was—he was . . . trespassing? And then, um, and then my dad went outside and slept in his car. And then my little brother jumped into my mum's bed. And then my dad came and started punching her in the neck? And then he just left without saying sorry or anything."

Articulate as she is, Mila is unlikely to use the word "vulnerable" to describe herself. Her stories, though, explain her silent appearances by my side. She has had a lifetime of vulnerable experiences. But Mila's vulnerability is interconnected with her mother's—her illness, her victimization by Mila's father—and this creates the context for Mila's vulnerability. Mila is dependent on her mother's care but also sees herself as essential to the care of her mother—an example of what the psychological literature terms "parentification," in which children take on parental roles within the family system (Broszormenyi-Nagy and Spark 1973). Several of her siblings have moved in with an adult sister, but Mila wants to stay with her mother so "I can look after her." Mila is frightened for her mother's safety, but she is also worried that if her father perceives that she is taking on too much of the care for the household, he will take her away from her mother, as has happened twice before. As the children understand, illustrated in chapter 5, children are not meant to be "parentified" and responsible for a parent's care, even if they sometimes need to be. In this way Mila's child status makes her twice vulnerable; her father's perception of her vulnerability means if she cares for her mother she may be taken away. Yet if she does not protect her mother, her mother's illness means that Mila may lose her anyway.

Like many of the other children I interviewed, Mila had internalized the warnings of the rheumatic fever campaign and showed a hypervigilance about sore throat. She estimated that she had visited the clinic twelve times that year, not because she experienced a sore throat but just to check, "to watch out for it, just in case I get it." Her sense of vulnerability was in part constituted by her perception of the risk of rheumatic fever, as conveyed through the frightening advertising. But unlike most others, she did not articulate her fear of sore throat in terms of her own illness or death, but because "my mum will worry."

"Your mum will worry?" I ask.

Mila explains, "and then, she'll like, take me to the doctor and everything, and then, I'll tell her that it's fine? And she'll be like, no, it ain't, you're sick! This ain't a fine thing to think about. And then, I'll go, ohhhh. And then, my mum says don't 'ohhh' yourself, 'cause you know that it's something to worry about."

Hearing her mother's concern about the possibility of her illness, Mila hears that her own vulnerability makes her mother vulnerable. In response, Mila goes to the clinic to get checked.

Mila also protects her mother in other ways. When her mother gets out of bed to do a chore and groans in pain, Mila will tell her mother to lie back down, and Mila will do the chore herself. And Mila tries to protect her mother from her father:

"I always watch them, like, every five minutes, I'll always walk into the room and say 'Hi! Hi! Hi!' And then they'll say, 'Can you please go out,' and I'll be like, 'OK.' And then, I'll walk out, and then I'll stand next to the door? And like, listen? And, if they're yelling I'll walk into the room and tell them to stop yelling."

On the day of our interview, Mila had been checked with the rest of her class through the class check that happens twice per term. She tells me, "I'm so lucky that the throat lady, she came around? And she came to our class. And she said that I was fine."

"Today?" I clarify. "How did you feel when she said you were fine?"

"I felt really happy, 'cause I knew that I was looking after myself really well."

Like many of the children, Mila attributed the origin or prevention of sore throat to her self-care, rather than parental care or social factors such as overcrowding. I asked her about the things she does to look after herself and keep her from getting a sore throat. Mila tells me she drinks lots of water and makes sure nothing bad happens to her.

"Like, making sure that nothing bad happens to you like what?" I ask.

"Like getting kidnapped, or . . . or like . . . getting murdered, or getting killed in my sleep."

I laugh because I think she is saying preventing these things will help prevent sore throat. But maybe Mila is saying that. In a world that includes gang conflict, schoolyard aggression, and the domestic assaults of relatives, maybe the threat of violence by illness becomes conflated with the threat of human violence.

Children's Bodies as Lenses for Vulnerability and Resilience

The practices of resilience that Mila has carved out for herself are bodily practices; she uses the presence of her body to diffuse tension between her parents and takes care of her physical health, drinking water and using the clinic to maintain her physical health to protect herself and her mother and find greater security. Her vulnerability is also embodied in her vigilant attention to her throat and the quiet moments when she stands with me and watches her world. These embodied practices parallel the more cognitive processes highlighted in cultural research with young adults; these children didn't express their resilience conceptually or in mantras or concepts, but it can be read in other languages nonetheless to shed light on where children feel insecure (Andresen 2014) and how they respond. Attention to embodied practices of resilience can also capture local norms of risk and resilience—norms that may be distinct in children's peer cultures from those of adults in the same community. These are culturally and ecologically derived ways of using bodies to protect, defend, and move forward in life.

Embodiment as a "lens" for reading vulnerability and resilience is appropriate given the centrality of the body in children's lived experience. Children's experience of their bodies is one of continuous growth and development, in which universal developmental trajectories are overlaid with cultural meaning. In the West, an emphasis on the "becoming" child means children's development is very much at the center of adult attention. Adults measure children's growth and keep a running commentary on changes, and hence events such as losing teeth and mastering new physical skills are chronicled by children themselves in recognition of their cultural significance (James 1993). Children's bodies are also a major component of their vulnerability; smaller, younger, or weaker children hold less physical power than those who are bigger, older, or stronger. This biological immaturity is used as the justification for "protections" that become embedded in social organization and policy in the form of segregation, restraints, and regulation but often limit children's agency and reinforce their dependency and lack of power (Mayall 1994; Qvortrup 1994). Becoming bigger, stronger, and more adult-like may be desirable as a pathway to greater autonomy and power, although growth is viewed in tension with the desire to be "normal" as determined by comparison with others in the same age group (James 1993). Being too big, as well as too small, can create additional vulnerability via self-consciousness and teasing or exclusion from peers.[4]

Hence the body is central to children's experience of vulnerability, and so its development and mastery is key to outmaneuvering insecurity.[5] However, the forms that children's bodily practices of resilience take may not match with clinical or even lay adult perspectives of what resilient functioning should look like. The recent shift toward culturally relevant conceptions of "doing well" troubles adult notions of what is in the "best interests" of children and is perhaps best illustrated by a burgeoning literature on the resourcefulness and well-being of street children (Mizen and Ofosu-Kusi 2013; Panter-Brick 2002). The spectrum of children's bodily practices includes a range of aggressive or violent behaviors that may be generally unsanctioned by adults in the community, but some of these behaviors may be considered normal or a form of resourcefulness by children themselves. These behaviors constitute what Ungar has termed "hidden resilience," or "culturally non-normative substitute adaptations" (Ungar 2011, 8). For example, a study of adolescent aggressive behavior in urban China found that a form of aggression termed "Ren Xing" was normalized and viewed as a functional strategy used by young women in Beijing to cope with culturally embedded gender bias in intimate relationships (Wang and Ho 2007). A culturally contextualized approach to processes of children's resilience may therefore need to consider children's practices not in terms of adult local cultural norms, but in terms of children's experiences, perspectives, and interpretations.

Children's Aggression as Accommodations for Resilience

Although proscribed by the New Zealand school system, for the children at Tūrama School, aggression is both a routine practice of self-protection and self-promotion and also a source of vulnerability for both perpetrators and those exposed. I do not think normalized forms of aggression are uncommon among children, nor specific to this context, although lower social tolerance for aggression in more recent times particularly among the middle class may have led to stricter monitoring in some schools. As described in chapters 2 and 3, while New Zealand law prohibits the use of any physical force toward children, talk of "getting a hiding" was pervasive at Tūrama School, and children's talk reflected a world where violence was normalized, integrated into play, and even a form of resourcefulness. As in the example of Ren Xing, the form this violence takes can often be distinctly gendered. For boys, in particular, aggression offered a strategy for navigating the vulnerabilities produced in this social world, while among girls, aggression toward others could be antisocial, and some girls established practices of harming themselves instead. In employing such practices to cope with their vulnerability, therefore, children can sometimes place themselves or others into new positions of risk. This does not mean that the tactics are not successful, just that successful coping in one domain of life may be at the expense of another.

Following Catherine Panter-Brick (1998a), I borrow from the human growth literature a way of conceptualizing this dimension of children's practices that acknowledges the realities of human practices of coping. While the term "adaptations" is used to describe a beneficial response to poor environments, the term "accommodations" was proposed as an alternative to draw attention to the costs and benefits of coping (Frisancho 1993). This reframing of survival in terms of "trade-offs" challenged the "small but healthy" view of stunted growth that was used to justify inaction in response to the chronic malnutrition of global populations. If resilience, or thriving despite adversity, represents a parallel to beneficial adaptation of biological systems, then accommodation represents a more accurate conceptualization of the many social processes that play out in the space between vulnerability and resilience. Practices of "navigating and negotiating resources," while effective, nonetheless often come at a cost. This has been noted by other researchers; Panter-Brick describes "entrapment," in which cultural values can be a double-edged sword when individuals struggle to conform to "what makes an honourable Afghan" (2012, 383) or when cultural values constrain or become maladaptive, for example when individuals cannot draw support from relatives because they cannot afford the expected reciprocal hospitality. Nancy Scheper-Hughes (2008) describes different "tactics of resilience," which she illustrates with ethnographic examples from families in shantytown Brazil and revolutionaries in apartheid South Africa. While some of these tactics might be celebrated as demonstrating the strength of vulnerable people in overcoming adversity, Scheper-Hughes notes other tactics might be seen as problematic or, as she diplomatically puts it, may "offend 'our' sensibilities and tastes, shaped by very different subjectivities, notions of value, human worth, and the good life, meaning always, the life that is worth living" (2008, 43). These tactics include normalization, such as maternal acceptance of a child's death; tactics of daily improvisation such as using trickery, cunning, or manipulation; "getting away with murder"; and socialization for toughness.

Hence, the responses of the children at Tūrama School may be viewed as accommodations to their circumstances—the responses of active agents within the structures of their ecological system, but responses that constrain options, produce new forms of vulnerability, or are simply seen as undesirable by those with more power, namely, adults. This is the case with aggressive or violent behavior, a protective strategy particularly used by boys in the context of peer relationships but often accompanied by adult sanction, risk of injury, and a loss of educational opportunities.

Nine-year-old Harrison described for me how he had been "the funniest and annoyingest in my class" as he entertained his classmates with amusing noises, but also how his teacher would have to restrain him when he got angry, like when "someone was like trying to be, like, being a dick to me and that . . . and

I was going to kick him in the head, which I did." Harrison was diagnosed with attention deficit hyperactivity disorder (ADHD) and anger management problems, suspended for three days, and according to him, eventually expelled. Observing Harrison's entry into playground life as the new boy at Tūrama School, I could imagine how he had come to settle on this aggressive strategy for survival; slightly built, freckled, and one of only three Pākehā boys in the senior school, his fair skin and light hair immediately marked him as a target for bullying.

One afternoon, while sitting on the mat, he showed me the injuries he'd acquired earlier at lunch, deep scratches on his arms and a scrape where he'd fallen down. He was aroused, talking quickly, clearly still intoxicated by a cocktail of adrenaline and pride. A week later in our interview, he tells me about the incident: how he'd gotten into a fight with another boy, Kyrone, because Harrison had "amped him up." We are in the school library, drawing sharks at a table, but now Harrison stands up, physically retelling the altercation.

"I kicked him in the head, I punched him. Oh no, I punched him there, I went dah!" He swings at an imaginary Kyrone. "And then he got angry, kicked me there, kicked me in the muscle . . . like this bit?" He lifts his leg and points.

"In the calf?" I clarify.

He nods. "In the calf, and then, um, punched me there, like there," he points to his jaw and chest. "And a knuckle went there, and then I got pissed off and kicked him in the head. I kicked him in the head twice."

I ask if he got in trouble when this happened, but Harrison isn't finished.

"I . . . ah, he like, when I kicked him in the head? I went like that, and then I fell on this side and then scraped my leg, down here?"

"Mm, I remember."

"And then I had to go to the sick bay. And Miss, the one, the old teacher at room eight? Now she's at room fifteen? Yeah, she's like—" he pants, hyperventilating. "And then she's, like, 'Wow, your heart is beating like a cheetah!'" He laughs. "Yeah, and I'm like—" he gasps for breath. "I was angry and that."

In describing this incident, Harrison positions himself not as a victim of bullying, but as the instigator of the fight, who "amps up" Kyrone, initiates the first kick, and deals the final blows. He catalogs each moment of the fight, his injuries, and the experience of his bodily responses, the racing heartbeat and ragged breathing. He was an active participant in the fight and is active in its recall. In this incident, he contested his vulnerability and won. Through his aggressive tactics, Harrison rejects victimhood; he is decidedly invulnerable, he is resilient.

Harrison is not the only boy to employ these aggressive practices of resilience, but they come at a cost. As well as risking physical injury, Harrison was regularly in trouble with his old school, and his behavior may have improved his standing with his peers but was incompatible with academic success. While Harrison had thus far evaded sanction for his behavior at Tūrama School, other boys found themselves habitually in trouble, and I would regularly see the deputy principal walking across the school trailed by those who had been sent to him that day. Several boys were suspended during my time at Tūrama School for up to three days. As an accommodation for resilience, aggression could be a successful and culturally accepted strategy within the peer ecology, but it caused difficulties when conflicting with adult standards of behavior and academic discipline.

Self-Harm: A Symptom or a Practice of Resilience?

Aggressive behavior such as Harrison's is one variable that would typically define "negative outcomes" in a dimension of "prosocial" behaviour often used as a measure of resilience in traditional research. This kind of research has been criticized for the implication that individuals who do not exhibit the "positive" behavior are not resilient, as measured by an ethnocentric social standard. In fact, a closer perspective might reveal behavior such as aggression to be functional in specific domains and therefore indicative of an individual who has adapted to their circumstances in a way that works for the individual. Likewise, it has been suggested that while dropping out of school is often seen as a "negative outcome," for some marginalized young people, this can be an adaptive strategy to sustain social well-being (Dei 1997). Yehuda and Flory (2007) also argue that PTSD symptoms, the absence of which has long been used as a marker of resilience, can be experienced by people who nonetheless show great resilience in their capacity to cope with symptoms. PTSD symptoms might actually indicate resilience when successfully managed, rather than being a sign of less resilient functioning. All of these examples point to issues with definitions of resilience that rely on normative assumptions about pathology and adaptation.

In the same way that PTSD symptoms are constructed as indicators of pathology in biomedical models of distress, self-harm is another phenomenon that would be considered a "symptom" of "non-resilient functioning" in much resilience research. Instead, I argue that self-harm could be seen as another example of an embodied practice of resilience, at least in this context. "Self-harm" is the most recent in a revolving door of terminology[6] describing deliberate, self-inflicted injury such as cutting, burning, breaking bones, poisoning, branding, scratching and picking at skin, or pulling out hair. The term, which often eludes clinical definition, excludes "socially sanctioned" injury such as piercing or tattoos, or harmful behavior such as smoking or excessive alcohol consumption, and precludes suicidal intent. Traditionally the purview of clinical fields, self-harm is still not well understood from psychological perspectives, which have tended to characterize the behavior as histrionic or stemming from poor impulse control (Steggals 2015). The inclusion of nonsuicidal self-injury disorder (NSSID) in the latest edition of the Diagnostic and Statistical Manual of Mental Disorders (DSM-V) (American Psychiatric Association, 2013)—not yet as a formal diagnosis, but under the conditions for further study with proposed diagnostic criteria[7]—nonetheless represents the next step in attempts to medicalize the phenomenon within a clean, clinical box.

Recently, sociologists have turned their attention to self-harm, unpacking behaviors like cutting not in terms of a natural and timeless category of illness but as an embodied, socially constructed phenomenon that is partially constituted by the psychological discourses that pathologize it (Adler and Adler 2011; Steggals 2015). While evidence of self-injurious behavior is found throughout history, Steggals argues that the past two decades have seen the rise of a particular and novel form of self-harm, a heterogeneous psychopathology that has been produced out of punk/emo-era bodily expressions of transgression and disenfranchisement, as well as a medical framing that reinforces self-harm as a socially recognized idiom of distress. In other words, self-harm is a mental health issue because society historically said it was a mental health issue, and self-harm has now become the quintessential expression of mental suffering, a "signifying wound" that takes a "distinct and recognisable form in our contemporary cultural language" (2015, 1–3).

The prevalence of self-harm among children under twelve is not known in New Zealand, although the behavior has been increasing among adolescents. Recent years have seen what has been described as an "epidemic" of self-harm in Aotearoa, with 29.1 percent of girls and 17.9 percent of boys in the most recent National Youth Health Survey of secondary school students (approximately ages twelve through eighteen) reporting that they had deliberately hurt themselves in the past twelve months, up from 26 percent and 15.5 percent, respectively, in 2007 (Fleming, Clark, Denny, et al. 2014). This is a particularly high rate when compared with rates in other countries (Muehlenkamp, Claes, Havertape, et al. 2012), but mirrors the gender difference found in other studies, which early feminist analyses suggest reflect the result of gendered socialization to externalize or internalize anger (Adler and Adler 2011). At Tūrama School, self-harm was also a gendered practice, although I am not fully aware of its extent. I came to know of groups of girls in at least three classrooms, but in general this was a secretive practice that was known to other children but kept hidden from adults. Like some of the teachers, I caught glimpses when walking the line between the adult and child worlds, but it was a very partial view.

When Skylar comes to hug me and won't let go, telling me she's sad about other children teasing her about liking a boy, we wander into a conversation about shaving body hair and she tells me she cut herself with a razor and then shows me her scars. Soraya was more direct, saying, "Look, Julie," before showing me the cuts on her arm. When playing paddle ball with Skylar's friend

Kaiyah, I catch sight of rows of parallel scratches and bruising on her arm, and when I ask about it she tells me she cuts herself. She runs off, but returns a little later, pointing to the bruises and asking me, "What is this?"

"Bruises?" I ask.

"No," she replies.

"Well how did you get them?" I ask.

"From sucking like this" she says, and demonstrates, twisting her arm to her mouth.

"Oh, hickeys?" I say.

"Oh, yeah, that's it," and she runs off again.

The next day I go to their classroom after lunch to check if their teacher is aware of what is going on. The children are lined up outside their classroom and, seeing me, they call out and swing on the rail, leaning over to hug me or talk (Figure 7). "Look at this, Julie," says Skylar, and shows me a long line of bruises on her arm. Kaiyah joins us and shows me hers. I rub Kaiyah's arm and ask if anyone else knows about it. Kaiyah whips her arm away. "No, don't tell anyone!"

She is whining, begging me not to tell. "I have to," I say.

"No! CYFs will take me away. They'll think I'm being abused!"

"They won't think you're being abused," I say gently. "They'll think you're unhappy at home."

"I am unhappy at home," she says matter-of-factly. "But they'll take me away from my brother. They'll take me away from my brother and I'm the only person he's got. I don't want to go without my brother."

Self-harm is often described as a private or covert practice. But in this new iteration it is also, even when done in secret, a social practice, in which feelings are experienced beyond the capacity of language to describe them and translated into a culturally recognizable, embodied expression of suffering. Kaiyah came to me seeking a label for her self-inflicted bruises, presumably not for her own personal knowledge but so that they could be talked about and understood as distinct from accidental bruising. Soraya shared her wounds with me directly, telling me something she couldn't express through language. In a world where adults may minimize or normalize children's experiences of bullying and powerlessness, and conceptualize children as resilient and adaptable, it may be difficult for children to be heard in any other way.

When questioned by teachers, the girls said they were upset over a boy, and this became the accepted reason behind what tended to be seen as a "fad" or attention-seeking. While it may be true that some were upset about a boy, this does not explain why groups of girls across at least three different classes took up cutting at around the same time. Knowing the stories of the girls involved—including experiences of bullying, intervention by CYF, and living with hostile, alcoholic, or abusive caregivers, not to mention other vulnerable experiences not recognized or validated by adults—it seems more likely that the story about a

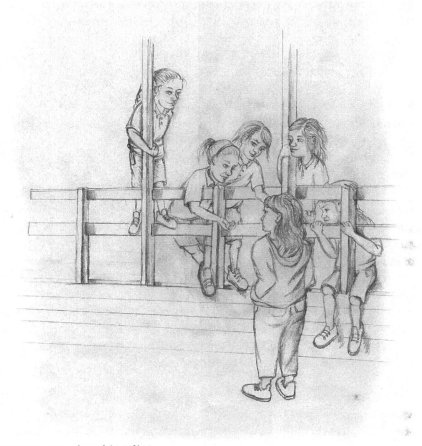

FIGURE 7 "Look at this, Julie."

boy was simply an easy answer to questioning authorities. And while some of the girls may have been "copycatting," as one teacher suggested, Adler and Adler (2011) point out that the documented "social contagion" of self-injury represents the transformation of self-harm into a recognized, demedicalized social practice symbolizing shared experience and social cohesion.

In its appearance as a sociological phenomenon, this form of self-harm does not easily fit with psychiatric models of a disorder of the troubled individual. Indeed, Adler and Adler (2011) found a growing Internet community who espoused perspectives ranging from acceptance and normalizing to embracing self-harm as a lifestyle choice or legitimate coping strategy that enabled functioning and represented a positive alternative to suicide. Wilkinson and Goodyer (2011) also point out problems with one of the DSM-V criteria, which require the nonsuicidal self-injury (NSSI) to be causing clinically significant distress or interference across different domains of functioning, noting that this requirement excludes large numbers of adolescents reporting NSSI because they tend to report their self-harm as helpful rather than distressing. This perspective on self-harm makes sense given that the practice may accompany suicidal thoughts but is qualitatively different, in that most people who self-harm do not wish to die but use self-harm as a tool to alleviate anxiety, stress, or low moods.

Instead, self-harm may be viewed as practice of resilience—one that may not fit with adult ideas about what children should be doing but is nonetheless functional in the way it makes invisible suffering visible. A practice that is socially sanctioned within the subcultures that foster it, self-harm enables that suffering to be expressed, shared, and validated. Viewing self-harm as a practice of resilience also illustrates how resilience is built upon accommodations: self-harm improves functioning in some domains or in the short term but at the cost of new vulnerabilities, the physical risks of injury and infection or the social impacts of scarring, stigma, and unwanted or negative attention. In this case, the school intervened and, unsure about what approach to take, initiated a chain of responses: involving the school social worker, contacting the families, and in the words of one teacher, explaining the behaviour as "very naughty little girls" who were only wanting attention and playing copycat.[8] From a social ecology that created certain experiences of vulnerability, children were able to generate their own practice for coping, but a practice that was quickly closed off by adults, with little recognition of the conditions that had produced this practice or the potential need for alternatives to fulfill the same function.

Conclusion

This chapter has analyzed children's vulnerability and resilience within a socio-ecological framework that acknowledges both children's agency and competency, and the environments that produce children's vulnerability and constrain their opportunities. This ethnographic perspective suggests a shift in the lens through which socio-ecological approaches view resilience to include specific dimensions of resilience practices—coproduction, interconnectedness, and accommodations—and with the body as an important locus through which these processes can be traced.

Using social networks to illustrate, I emphasize that children do not enter an environment that pre-exists them but instead actively coproduce that environment. As children like Ruby and Harrison experience the instability of relationships or direct threat of bullying, they exercise their agency in the form of strategic practices—the control of or aggression toward peers. Crucially, these practices shape the social environment, opening up new resources or creating new vulnerabilities that are experienced and negotiated by other children in turn. This interconnectedness of vulnerabilities and practices of resilience, seen also in the mutually constituting vulnerability of Mila and her mother, is a dimension of resilience that may be difficult to account for outside of ethnographic inquiry.

All of the children whose stories I tell in this chapter demonstrate resilience in different ways and in step with shifting circumstances they have little control over, but all of their practices of resilience vary in their success and incur costs; they are accommodations to their circumstances. Cassidee, who avoids fostering connections with peers she knows she may soon leave, misses out on the protective benefits that close relationships can bring. The tight control Ruby holds over her friends places children outside of the group into more vulnerable positions while offering resources to those within. Mila devotes great energy to vigilant attention to her body and to her mother's care. Other behaviors here that I have recognized as practices of resilience belong to that category of "atypical" resilience (Ungar, Brown, Liebenberg, et al. 2007) that would be instead labeled as "risks," "symptoms," or "negative outcomes" by traditional resilience research. These too incur costs, but while Harrison's aggressive behavior compromised his ability to succeed academically at school and put him at risk of injury, it also allowed a sense of agency, autonomy, and self-efficacy he might not otherwise be able to access in this context. The self-harm practiced by many girls at Tūrama School cost them in terms of the disciplinary action taken by the school and the risk of unintended injury but also gave them a sense of solidarity and social cohesion through partaking in this collective bodily expression that was likely protective, at least temporarily. The nature of resilience practices appears to vary by gender, as strategies such as aggression have gendered implications—in this case, while it is more acceptable among peers for boys express aggression toward others, girls are more likely to turn violence toward themselves.

This view of resilience practices is particularly relevant when considering how adults might resource children to support their resilience. Resources provisioned for the purpose of protecting children might be co-opted into strategies of resilience by some, contributing to a shift in the social ecology, which then opens up or constrains new resources or vulnerabilities. The clinic intervention, for example, appears to function as a catalyst for children's coproduction of a new, collective vulnerability, one that plays out for some in hypervigilant self-care practices and for others in denial or avoidance. Although this is a small ethnographic slice of life, the dimensions identified here—coproduction, interconnectedness, accommodations, and embodiment—could point to useful future pathways for the large-scale, mixed-method studies currently leading resilience research.

8

Talking with Death

Sitting around at our desks three weeks into the school year, I work quietly correcting spelling while listening to the chatter of the mixed-gender group of children around me. In general I found children's conversation hard to capture: frenetic and stuttering, multiple threads tangling across one another, and individuals, catching words from the breeze, abandon one line of conversation to chase another, mouths fighting to describe a connection only their mind has made. As such, the chatter of children can sound like an incoherent layering of disparate ideas, interruptings, and mumblings, a hubbub that is disregarded until it intrudes on adult conversation. Christensen describes how she had to develop an ability to "listen attentively" to children and not be distracted by the interruptions of others when in a group (1999, 75). Likewise, I found that I easily "tuned out" children's talk in such situations, since the conversation required a special effort to listen to and often lost me along the way.

On this day, the conversation clarified for a few moments around a particular topic that captured everyone's attention: What are you scared of? The answers fought to impress: aliens, crocodiles, snakes. I noticed with interest that the things named were not things that the children had any real experience with. "I'm not scared of anything," came one boast.

"You'd be scared if your mum died," came the retort. There was general agreement; a parent dying was a scary thought.

Childhoods in Aotearoa are not homogenous, and the degree to which death appears in childhood, both in fantasy and in reality, will likely vary alongside children's conceptions of death. For children at Tūrama School encounters with death are common. For many who are Māori, wide whānau connections mean that journeys to the marae for *tangi*, or funerals, are frequent, often extending three or four days at a time and, for many children, experienced as a holiday

(Jacob 2011). For the Pasifika children, too, the passing of relatives may mean a trip to the islands, to Tonga, where funerals are a preeminent social occasion and key locus for enculturation of the young (Kaeppler 1978), or to Samoa, where the dead stay alongside the living in front-yard graves (Havea 2013). In Auckland, too, family homes may be converted into "little marae" for Māori (Gagné 2013) and Pasifika lives celebrated with ritual even more traditional than in the home islands (Havea 2013).

Many children at Tūrama School also experienced the death of a close relative, including five children who lost a parent during my study period. Often, these children would quietly disappear from school as they were re-homed with whānau in another part of the city, leaving behind classmates who named what had happened with wide eyes and reverent voices. These children are socially marked, spoken of with hushed voices and respectful distance. They have experienced the far edge of child vulnerability, that place spoken of in fear across the classroom desks. That vulnerability is found in not just the daunting grief of the loss of parent, but also the social upheaval that follows for a child who must start a new life not of their choosing.

Child death frequently appears in ethnography, in which childhood mortality often forms the backdrop to ethnography of poverty-stricken or war-torn communities—the "unnaturalness" of child death used to emphasize the direness of conditions through statistics or vignettes. Nancy Scheper-Hughes's (1993) ethnography of shantytown Brazil paints a community so saturated with child death as to cleave the most primal bonds of mother and infant. Yet children's experiences of the death of their siblings, or their own close brushes with mortality, remain outside of the picture.

Only a small library of anthropological works represent the perspectives of children themselves on death. Significant works by Myra Bluebond-Langner (1978, 2000) have focused on chronically or terminally ill children in a North American context, demonstrating how children acquire knowledge of their prognosis or come to understand that their sibling will die. Based on research in Dehli, Veena Das (1989, 2015) reflects on the experiences and expressions of children who have witnessed violent deaths or coped with the loss of a parent. Ross Parsons (2012) combines psychotherapeutic and anthropological understandings to write of the ambivalent liminality of HIV-positive children enduring poverty in "the waiting room of death" in Zimbabwe. From different corners of the world, these scholars trace the way that death shapes the social world that children live in, just as it is shaped by adult notions of how children's encounters with death should be managed. Yet, for the most part, death in this literature is represented as an anomaly, even when common, undermining normal, carefree childhoods and leaving children to embroider its extraordinary tragedy in repetitive symbolic or embodied expressions. With the exception of Das's

(2015) portrait of a child renegotiating changes to the family structure as a result of illness and death, these are portrayed as transgressive deaths, not a death that touches childhood in the everyday.

The limited explorations of death in everyday childhood perhaps reflects what scholars have claimed to be a denial or general suppression of death in contemporary Western culture (Becker 1973; Ariès 1981), where despite a near-saturation of the media with death imagery, personal experiences of death are kept hidden or "invisible" and marked as taboo. This death, James Green (2012) adds, is seen as particularly inappropriate for children, whose lives are meant to be innocent and happy, free from adult burdens. Once commonplace, over the past century death has come to be seen as out of place in children's everyday in the recent West (Kastenbaum and Fox 2008), viewed as a threat to the social order (Bluebond-Langner 1978). This is well illustrated by the "mutual-pretense" of Bluebond-Langner's (1978) dying children and their parents: planning Christmases that would never arrive, continuing with school, and maintaining the socialization of the child for an adulthood that all knew would not come. Discussions of death and childhood therefore often begin with the Western premise that death ought not to be part of children's lives, analyzing the way adults and children alike make sense of this anomaly.

However, death is part of children's everyday lifeworlds, although their personal experiences of death can be limited. From children's films, where death is seen 2.5 times as often as in adult films (Colman, Kingsbury, Weeks, et al. 2014), to religious stories, to violent toys and video games, to classroom discussions (at Tūrama School, a full term on World War I), death is already central to children's cultural systems, structuring everyday meaning and practices and enacted through play. Pioneering studies by Nagy (1948) and Anthony (1972) in early psychology showed that death-related phenomena often appear in children's thinking within their everyday lives, and children had their own questions and theories. For Māori and Pasifika children, the presence of death in the everyday is even more overt, and their personal experiences of death more frequent than for their Pākehā contemporaries. What role then, does death play, and what meanings do children construct from death in the everyday?

Small Talk of Death

I did not set out to learn about children's perspectives on death. I did not raise death as a question in the interviews I held after school with children, parents, or teachers, and I did not explore children's experiences of tangi. However, I found that my field notes, interviews, and even children's drawings were saturated with references to death—unsurprising, given the proximity of death in these children's lives, and revealing of the salience and relevance of death to childhood. Children cataloged, memorialized, and constructed relationships with the dead; concocted understandings of the afterlife; and experimented with mortality through risk. I cannot offer here a child ontology of death, or comment on their understandings and knowledges of death—a topic that has been considerably discussed within psychology and counseling fields (e.g., Anthony 1972; Cuddy-Casey and Orvaschel 1997; Nagy 1948). Instead, this is an analysis of the way that death is woven into the discourses and practices of everyday life outside of death events and rituals, the appearance of death in life's little conversations, and what this can tell us about childhoods lived in the classroom, at the kitchen table, on the playground. This differs from studies that set out to ask about death, and instead stumbles across the ways that death creeps unsummoned into everyday childhoods.

In children's "small talk of death"—how children express death and how children use death to express other things—can be found the social meanings children construct around death, but also the experience of childhoods as shaped by broader political, economic, and social forces. As such, I argue that the meanings of death for children are shaped by their social position as children, a possibly universal process of apprehending this intriguing idea that existences will end, coupled with a structural vulnerability that inoculates the interpretations of those unknowable deaths with threat of social displacement. However, concepts of death are also colored by the particularities of children's social circumstances, and so, for the children at Tūrama School, their death talk also reflects plural cultural frames and a structural violence that mediates their experience of death. Children's understandings of death are shaped by their experience of life, and so children's death talk can also function as a window for understanding childhood.

As co-constructors of their own cultures but also embedded within adult worlds, the way children appropriate and reproduce their own versions of death can be usefully conceptualized through William Corsaro's (1992) model of interpretive reproduction, in which children spin their own webs of meaning over the scaffolding of adult institutions. As described in chapter 1, Corsaro breaks away from theories of socialization that position the child as individually and privately acquiring the skills, knowledge, and culture of adults, instead viewing childhood socialization as a collective, social process, occurring within peer cultures as much as with adults, and reproductive rather than linear. My analysis, therefore, begins in children's peer talk, where snippets of experience are collectively patchworked.

Death in Cultural and Structural Context

Eleven-year-old Arya is eager to be interviewed, and as soon as I turn on the recorder she begins talking and doesn't stop, one thought tumbling into another, punctuated with bright-eyed laughter and the rising inflection common of Kiwi cadence. She begins by telling me about her family's history of gang violence, but her stream of consciousness leads into a cataloging of deaths in her family, a theme she keeps returning to annotate again and again.

"And then my cousin, he wanted to give the Crips gang a hiding, but they told him that they should just leave us alone? We had, like, bad people in our family? That got rushed—my cousin got . . . beaten last week? And my papa died the year before, like 2012? And our papa died? Well my other papa died on my dad's side, ages ago, I think it was 2010? And it was heartbreaking because he was a good cooker and—and—we loved him and we gave him everything, like he wanted?"

Disoriented by the shift in topic, I ask, "Did he die because of the gangs?"

"Oh, no, he died because he had a back injury. Oh, sore back."

"He died from a sore back?"

"And he was sick," she adds and continues, "that's the same as my little sister. She's like, eight now, and she passed away in 2007. And my cousin, oh, we had a big-as tangi and funeral? Because everyone liked her, and my auntie, that was her—that was her godmother? And that's the one that—she loves me, now? But she still—she still loves her, like her daughter, like she wants her to be her daughter? And—and my family was so sad. And that was my little sister, she's— she turned eight, in . . . April. On the twenty-third."

"Do you guys do anything for her birthday?"

"Yes, we went to go clean her grave and put flowers and stuff. And . . . we sing—sometimes sing a song to her. When we go past."

Later in the interview Arya returns to her topic, adding further infant deaths that occurred before she was born and the death of another papa in 2014. The way children like Arya talked about the deaths of their relatives echoes some universal fascinations with the nature of existence and its cessation, the continuation of relationships after death, and some specific features of childhood. However, children's death talk is also shaded with the particularities of their circumstances, which add the nuance of experience. For children at Tūrama School, these particularities include a structural violence that burdens whānau with earlier and more frequent death. In addition, these are children of plural and syncretic cultures, who incorporate multiple frames of death into their own understandings. Children experience, for example, the way that Western medicalized frames of death shape everyday life into a series of risk preventions (McIntosh 2001), from road-crossing patrols at school, to legislation mandating child-resistant closures on medications and chemicals. Likewise, Westernized medical institutions invoke death in the management of illness, which Tūrama School children absorb through health promotion warnings about the deadly threat of rheumatic fever. Meanwhile, many of these children, predominantly of Māori and Pasifika descent, have grown up in cultures where death is not out of place in children's lives; dying is not cordoned off into hospitals, nor is old age.

Instead, death is axial to life, the boundaries between living and dead blurred, and children themselves may be considered intermediaries to the spirit world (Counts and Counts 1985; Gagné 2013; Metge 1967).

For example, care and connections with the dead are infused throughout Te Ao Māori, or the Māori world, and vice versa, as expressed by Māori writer Harry Dansey: "We cannot think of the dead without reference to the living" (1975, 174). The depth of relationship forged from shared, even ancient ancestry, is tied to a deep emotional expression for even those little known to the mourner (McIntosh 2001; Rosenblatt 2011; Sinclair 1990). Death is also embedded in the architecture of Māori social life, where marae, or traditional meeting places, are explicitly designed for the hosting of many visitors for *tangihanga* (funerals) (Gagné 2013; Salmond 1976). This centrality of tangi to Māori life is far from the "invisible death" that Philippe Ariès (1981) saw as marking contemporary Western cultures. Very little has been written about children's perspectives of tangi, although Jacob's (2011) research with Māori parents includes the recollections of adult participants who compare childhood experiences of attending tangi to going on holiday. For these Māori, tangi were not unusual but remembered as a break from the normal everyday grind, a chance to see relatives and play with cousins for days on end, free of adult responsibility and relatively unsupervised. Depending on the closeness of the deceased, the business of grieving could be secondary to the excitement of the trip and reunion with whānau. This was also a familiar experience for the Māori children of Tūrama School, and talk of attending tangi formed a part of everyday conversation.

Yet while culture makes meaning of the dead, encounters with death are also mediated by the structural. Living at the extreme end of socioeconomic disadvantage, Tūrama School children's experience of death is again amplified. To understand how death articulates with context here, I use the related concepts of structural violence and structural vulnerability. Commonly attributed to Johan Galtung (1969), structural violence is a concept used by anthropologists such as Paul Farmer (2003, 2004) and Nancy Scheper-Hughes (2004, 1996) to bring a critical perspective to health inequalities. Structural violence refers to the way that sets of historical and economic conditions, when protected as the status quo, result in physical or spiritual harm, disease, oppression, and premature death (Farmer 2003). While the effects of poverty, racism, or gender inequalities can be misrecognized as misfortune, structural violence conceptualizes systems—and the people who uphold them—as perpetrators of harm. Quesada and colleagues (2011) propose "structural vulnerability" as an extension of structural violence that explicitly includes cultural and idiosyncratic sources of structurally mediated distress, such as symbolic taxonomies of worthiness or discourses of normativity. Children, because of their perceived vulnerability, incompetence, and low status, are also rendered structurally vulnerable through society's adult-centric organization, often encoded in legislation, which separates them from the adult world, constraining their political power and limiting their voice (Frankenberg, Robinson, and Delahooke 2000).

The appearance of death in the cultural milieu of Tūrama School can be seen as both a reflection of a structural violence that mediates the degree of children's experience with death, and a structural vulnerability that produces a particular experience of childhood. As a result of economic inequities, institutional racism, and colonization, Māori death rates tend to be higher than those for non-Māori at all ages, although the gap is narrowing, and life expectancy at birth for Māori is about seven years lower than for non-Māori in New Zealand (Statistics New Zealand 2015). Pasifika peoples in New Zealand have life expectancy about 1.5 years higher than for Māori but still well below the rest of the population. Infant mortality rates are higher for Māori (0.65 percent) and Pasifika (0.62 percent) than for the general population (0.45 percent) (Statistics New Zealand 2015), and 2013 data show that the Māori suicide rate was 1.6 times higher than the overall population and that the Māori youth suicide rate was 3.1 times the rate for non-Māori (Ministry of Health 2016).

The experiences of the children living in the community surrounding Tūrama School reflect these statistics, and the death of a close relative was not uncommon. Aside from the passing of many grandparents during the study period, five children in my cohort (two of them brothers) lost parents to illness-related deaths. The deaths of each of these parents affected not only their children but also their nephews, nieces, and cousins attending the school. Some children disclosed personal knowledge of a relative who had died by suicide, while two ten-year-old boys described to me the phenomenon of suicide ideation in detail, suggesting great familiarity ("Like, having a bad life and everything has been . . . bad in their life, they could say, 'I want to kill myself.' Then change their mind and think about their family, and what that will do. And then they say, 'Oh, nah'"). For eleven-year-old Pikau, the ideation was a personal experience, as she disclosed to me how she had thought of killing herself after years of being bullied.

As well as the structural position of Māori and Pasifika which brings death earlier, the structural vulnerability of *children* in society gives these deaths special meaning. As in many Western countries, children in Aotearoa are one of the most legally and socially restricted groups in society, with limited mobility, political power, and earning ability. Although children's smaller body size leaves them more vulnerable than adults, their dependency in these contexts is to a large degree created by adults who are concerned with their care and protection. In other societies, even very young children can move independently through their community, access material resources, and care for one another in peer groups, rather than rely exclusively on adults. In some circumstances, street children, for example, can obtain better nutrition than children who live at home (Gross, Landfried, and Herman 1996), indicating that dependency on adult care is to a certain extent structural, rather than only biological. Children's near-complete dependence on adults in Aotearoa, therefore, is less about an innate vulnerability and more the product of their structural vulnerability in an adult-centric society that often marginalizes children.

Children's structural vulnerability has two implications relevant to this discussion of death. First, in rendering children so dependent on adults, the threat of death, particularly of a caregiver, represents a threat to the social life of the child. When parents fall ill or die, dependent children must be placed elsewhere in the whānau, a dislocation of relationships, home, and often school that can be a disorienting addendum to grief, even though children's belonging is more fluid in Pacific kinship than for Pākehā (Metge 1967; Morton 1996; Ritchie and Ritchie 1979). Second, the adult-centric distribution of power in society often means that children are invisibilized in culture and policy. Subsequently, children may be exploited for adult agendas, with little regard for what this means for children. This can particularly be seen in health promotion messaging that links children and medicalized, Pākehā frames of death in order to motivate parents but inadvertently influences children's conceptions of death and subsequent practices, as in the rheumatic fever campaign. The experience of structural violence and structural vulnerability for the children of Tūrama School can be observed through analyzing both how children express death and how they use death to express themselves in everyday life.

Expressing Death

At morning tea one day, I sit with Ruby and Soraya, our backs against the classroom wall at the edge of the playground. As we watch a group of girls and boys kicking a soccer ball around on the field, I tune in to their talk, which has taken on a somber tone. "My nephew died," says Soraya, gap-toothed and with a smile that curls up at the edges. "My little four-year-old nephew, you know? Because he wasn't eating anything."

"My cousin died," says Ruby, her eyes big.

"Everything he ate up, he threw up," Soraya continues. "Vegetables . . . meat . . ."

"—My cousin was 16," adds Ruby.

". . . lollies . . . everything, he threw up." A stray ball flies toward us, and Soraya intercepts it with the edge of her foot, booting it back toward the field.

"Did you know he was going to die?" Ruby asks.

"No," Soraya answers. "We didn't know he was sick until we took him to hospital. And then they sent him home, but then he died."

"My cousin hung herself," says Ruby. "That's really sad," I respond.

"Oh my god!" Soraya interjects. "That's the same—not the *same*, but that's the same thing as my little nephew. But he died in hospital. 'Cause he was getting fed the right things but he couldn't breathe when he ate it. Like every time he ate something, he would just stop breathing."

This "small talk of death" is woven through children's desktop chatter, in the sharing of global and personal news on the classroom mat, and in playground banter. These small conversations are where children engage in a process of collective bricolage, pooling their experiences of death to make sense of its place in their world. Ruby and Soraya "name" the whānau members who have died, an intensive cataloging of deaths that is usually accompanied by the manner of death, if known. Children often included dates in their catalogs and the age a sibling would be if still alive; Arya refers to her sister as "eight now." This is a sharing and comparing of experiences in order to apprehend death, but children also register who knows what by indexing who was affected ("Liam's mother died. And she was Trystan's auntie"). While I contribute a comment on the sadness of the death, as teachers tend to do, Ruby and Soraya do not talk about what feelings or meanings they associate with the death. Instead, they add to their catalog, a practice that takes on a tone of one-upmanship, using experience of death to compete and impress, and drawing comparisons; Ruby's cousin's death by hanging was "the same" as Soraya's nephew who couldn't eat. Claiming a close experience with death could thus function as a form of social capital, impressing others with the reminder of their vulnerability and the knowledge of something all children will experience at some point but that some have not yet faced. In an interview with two nine-year-old boys, I hear the following snippet of conversation:

WHETU: None of my family has ever died yet. Only my nan. My mum's mum.

JACKSON: My nan died two years ago.

WHETU: My nan died four years ago.

Rehearsing cultural scripts for talking about death through somber tones, in this talk children situate themselves in wider networks of relationships that continue after death. At the same time, the comparisons and repeated indexing of death also mark these deaths as a salient part of children's experience.

Children's expressions of death therefore express their experience of *life*, one where the deaths of family members echo with threats about those who *could* die. "Whose mums and dads died in this group?" one boy asked a group of classmates during a brainstorm of what it means to be a child. "If you're young, and your mum and dad die, who would you live with?"

"Your grandparents," another child replies.

"Yeah, your grandparents."

"Or your brother and sister if you have them. If they're older."

What it means to be a child, then, is to be dependent on networks of care for social survival.

Death in the Classroom

On the first day back from the spring holidays, after the usual Monday assembly, Mrs. Steven's class settles on to the mat to start the day. As is their routine, Mrs. Stevens asks, "What news do we have today?" The children scramble to name the local and global headlines they'd picked up over the holidays. New Zealand has made the quarter-finals of the Rugby World Cup, and evidence has been found of water on Mars. "Lots of murders," one child calls out.

"Yeah, that boy got murdered!"

"Yes, I think his funeral is today," Mrs. Stevens acknowledges. The disappearance and subsequent discovery of a ten-year-old's body in the South Island had captured the attention of the nation for the past week. "That boy was murdered, Julie," a girl said to me.

"A lady died while she was feeding her baby and her baby died, too!" another child adds, and Mrs. Stevens pulls open her laptop and finds the story from earlier that week. "How did she die, Miss?" children ask, and Mrs. Stevens reads from the article: "She collapsed and died of bronchitis."

"What's bronchitis?" Mrs. Stevens explains about infections in the bronchial tubes; this is how much of the learning happens in this class, through informal dialogue on the mat.

"My auntie died, Miss! Aye, Miss! Aye, my auntie died!" Eleven-year-old Trystan, who was lying on the ground, leaps to his feet (Figure 8).

"Oh, yes, she did," Mrs. Stevens realizes, meeting my eye.

"She died of new—pnew—pneumonia," Trystan wraps his tongue around the word. "She didn't go to the doctor."

"And she was Liam's mum!" Another child adds.

"What?" I hadn't noticed Liam's absence until that moment. Quiet and small, Liam had joined the class only a few months ago.

"Yeah, Liam's moved to Ferndale," Mrs. Stevens tells the class. Turning to me, she adds, "It's a shame he's not here so we could support him with his mum dying. He didn't want to leave Tūrama."

Death, then, makes a regular presence in the classroom, not only for these children who are directly affected by loss, but also for those around them who bear witness to and imagine as their own the experiences of their classmates and the boy in the newspaper. After rugby news, children tended to share the death stories, a cataloging of global deaths to mirror the real ones they encountered. But their structural vulnerability is brought into relief this day, when the death of Liam's mother was followed by his abrupt disappearance from the class he liked and the teacher who cared for him.

Trystan was clearly impacted by the death of his aunt, which he brought up with me on several other occasions. However, the expressions of children who had lost a parent were quieter; Teuila, tells me that her dad is—present

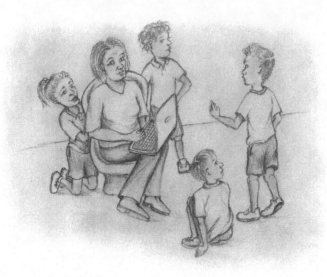

FIGURE 8 "My auntie died, Miss!"

tense—an artist who taught her to draw, and sits silently as her teacher reads to the class newspaper articles about his premature death. In my interview with Cassidee, I invited her to draw for me a picture illustrating either something she enjoyed doing at school or a time when she found things tough. She would not let me see her drawing in the interview, frantically covering it with her arms, and asking that I only look at it after she left. When I remembered to pull out the drawing a few days later, I found a depiction of her father's death (Figure 9).

Once death has struck so close, children's expressions turn away from its apprehension, and toward commemorating, memorializing, and configuring relationships with the dead.

Expressions of Death; Death as Expression

The way that the children of Tūrama School talk of death is consistent with how death is expressed by children in many other contexts in academic literature, where ethnographic vignettes show children engaging directly and expressively with death encounters. These expressions can often look quite different from those of adults in the same community; in the context of Tongan childhoods, for example, Morton describes the aftermath of the suicide of a neighbor boy, where adults were distressed and quiet, while "children were excitedly chattering, telling me the details of how he had been found, what his face looked like in death, how it was originally thought he must have been electrocuted, and how his mother was in deep shock, rocking on her bed and calling out to him as if

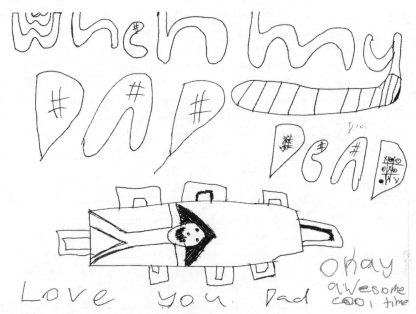

FIGURE 9 "When My Dad Died" by Cassidee, age ten. The gray writing is presumably referring to the experience of being interviewed.

he were still alive" (Morton 1996, 241–242). When adults began to recover from the shock, they discussed the death only briefly to agree on the motivations behind the suicide, before moving on to planning the funeral and positive recollections of the boy and his mother.

Likewise, among families of children with cystic fibrosis, Bluebond-Langer (2000) found that although parents and children rarely talked to each other about the prognosis, children's talk is littered with references to death, which increase as their sibling's condition progresses. While parents avoided thinking about or discussing the prognosis even as their child's condition deteriorated, children's talk belies a preoccupation with dying. However, children's expressions are not limited to the verbal. In her earlier work with terminal leukemia patients, Bluebond-Langer describes a proliferation of death imagery emerging after children came to understand that they were dying; a child who used to draw birds and flowers began to draw crucifixion scenes, another made only "turtles for people's graves" (1978, 185) and buried her paper dolls in tissue boxes, and cohorts of children asked to be read the chapter of *Charlotte's Web* in which Charlotte dies. Behaviorally too, children expressed their impending death, for example through a concern with the passage of time: admonishing parents not to "waste time" and becoming angry when people took "too long." Das (1989) also describes how Delhi children who witnessed anti-Sikh riots expressed the death of parents in embodied ways; one child mimes the hanging of his father, while others are haunted by nightmares of ghosts. Vivid and direct expressions of death are therefore found among children in many contexts where death has been experienced.

These vignettes are used to reveal children's knowledge of their or their sibling's prognosis, how children make sense of the death and violence they have witnessed, and how they draw together fragments of adult conversations to weave their own coherent narratives in a collective reconstructing of events and experiences. In unpacking Tūrama School children's references to death, it is apparent that children are not only expressing knowledge of death or fear or sadness, nor just engaging in a collective bricolage to make sense of this death concept. The children also spoke of death not in reference to death itself, but in order to invoke the connotations of death to express *other* experiences. Death is not only expressed but also used *to* express. So when Ruby and Soraya tell me that some people who are cyberbullied "get to, like, dying," they are telling me about the seriousness of cyberbullying, as well as the seriousness of death. When 11-year-old Navahn tells me about the gang his family are involved in, he tells me that "they have heaps of fights, they die," to convey the degree of violence. And when nine-year-old Hinemaia says strep throat "could stop you from breathing, and that could kill you too," she uses death to explain the threat of a sore throat. Children's talk of death, therefore, is important for what it says about life.

Expressing Illness with Death

Children's appropriation of death terminology to communicate ideas about other things can be most clearly seen in their expression of illness. The bundling of death with illness is in part because death in this community is often caused by illness, although death could also be used to convey ideas about bullying and violence, as described earlier. However, to speak about illness also requires a specific lexicon, one that children are still acquiring. By contrast, when parents speak of illness, the language employed is quite different from that of children. Anna, in telling me of her son Anton's illness history, draws from an extensive and nuanced language of sickness, acquired through her years of parenting experience. When Anton was born he was "meconium," "stressed because he was overdue," and "he wasn't breathing." She describes the efforts of the doctors, the effects on his throat and lungs, how his temperature of 40°C could lead to a seizure, and the work she did to steam his excess mucus. This is not a language that Anton shares. When he tells me about "one of my bad sickness," a spider bite, he tells me that his mum took him to the doctors and describes what the doctor said: "Your son got poisoned, but I don't think he's gonna like die or something, it's just like, you know, he's gonna be sick." He adds, "And my greatest fear was like, dying." After telling me about how the spider bite "restarted my memories" and ignited a new interest in soccer, Anton returns to the theme of death:

"I was in hospital just for the great white tail spider, but, lucky . . . he didn't said, 'You got a poisoning and you're gonna die.' Lucky he didn't said that. But he says he got a cure, and that. And then, he—he, like, had a needle put in my, like, I think like right here?"

"Oh, he put a needle in your side?"

"Yeah. And then right before, he said, 'You're not going to die.'"

Lacking the vocabulary of symptoms and treatment, Anton emphasizes his experience in terms of proximity to death—Anton feared he might die, but luckily the doctor said he wasn't going to die, such was the seriousness of his sickness. When I ask him why he was thinking about dying, he grapples for the words to express the experience of his body in that moment:

"It kind of felt like, I kinda feel like my heart—my heart beating was, like, like, slowing down . . . Wait, I was actually—I was actually ill, but—a little ill, so—it was still—it was, like, going slooooww . . . and then going faster and then going slow and then going faster. It's kind of . . . It's kind of scared. And, like, and I was, like, um . . . was my heart going to explode or something."

The language of death, therefore, can function for children as an effective shortcut to communicate the seriousness of an illness experience, a way that children can express and be understood by other children unfamiliar with the vocabulary of arrhythmia or anti-venom injections.

Similarly, death is the focus of the story of Te Rerenga's birth, as narrated by her and her sister Nga-Atawhainga in the middle of a discussion about illness experiences at their kitchen table. After asking her mother whether she had been sick as a baby, nine-year-old Nga announces:

"My sister nearly died when I was a baby."

"Yes, no, she had a struggle to life, Rere did," her mother Tūmanako agrees.

"She nearly died when she come out. Mum told us."

"How does that feel?" I ask eight-year-old Rere, whose face is ringed with chocolate from the cookies I brought.

"Like, the same," Rere answers, I think meaning she feels the same as she always does, that how she feels is not the important thing. She continues. "My mum nearly died when she got—"

"—Mum got a fever when I was having her," Tūmanako interjects, switching narrative perspective halfway through her sentence. While Rere attempts to continue, Tūmanako narrates a parallel story, this one told through symptoms and treatments and their effects.

"Oh, and I nearly died—"

"And then because we had an inexperienced person trying—"

"—I was sick when I was four or five—"

"—to give me an epidural, they nearly paralyzed me—"

"—when I was little you took me to the hospital—"

"—because you were too big to come out I had to have a cesarean section. I tried to tell them that, 'cause I'd been in labor for five hours, I was, like, 'Look, last time it only took me an hour for the whole thing, I'm telling you I can't do this, please listen, you're going to kill me,'" Tūmanako finishes, laughing. "She didn't have a good start to life, Rere."

Interestingly, as her daughters, lacking the language of labor and cesareans, refer repeatedly to death to convey to me the gravity of the event, Tūmanako's only reference to death is also deployed in another moment of misunderstanding. "You're going to kill me," she laughs now, but at the time communicated what Tūmanako's body knew but couldn't express in any other way to the "inexperienced" doctor.

With less experience of verbal communication, particularly the vocabulary associated with exceptional illness events, children therefore draw on their own categories of concepts to signify the most serious, the most frightening of events. Along with death, Anton and Rere both make reference to the hospital, another signifier of a serious medical condition. For the children at Tūrama School, the hospital is an important symbol of sickness, differentiating notable sickness from the everyday. In one lunchtime conversation, children discussed hospital visits, asking me how many times I'd been to hospital and calculating the times they went to hospital and their injuries.

The use of death language in their everyday talk therefore also speaks to what death means for children. Adults, with longer experience, may have more of a sense of life's rhythms than children, who are still calibrating their sense of death's relative frequency. Adults can suffer greatly in bereavement and face social disruption, but with their greater agency and autonomy are less socially threatened by the death of relatives than children are by the loss of caregivers. For children, death means the deepest and most insecure grief, as they are tossed into the waves of a social upheaval, with little control over where and with whom they may land.

Death Management in Health Promotion

Children's talk of death in this context reflects their own structural vulnerability, the structural violence that makes death a common occurrence in this community, and cultures that make meaning from those deaths. However, children's conceptions of death are also shaped by Pākehā medicalizations of death—how, as McIntosh (2001) describes, with the rise of modern technologies and medicines, mortality is deconstructed into a series of discrete problems, manageable through "taking control" of the body, adopting healthy practices and abstaining from the unhealthy. When death comes to be seen as solvable, then life becomes a series of risk preventions, as McIntosh puts it, "an attempt to write death small" (2001, 247) which paradoxically leaves death imprinted over life in seat belts and alarms and expiration dates. Public health campaigns fixate on death as the enemy, even when, as is the case with rheumatic fever, death is the least likely outcome. The effect of this fixation is to semiotically link illness to death; health care, even for children, becomes constructed in terms of death management.

"And what about cancer, what do you know about that?" I ask nine-year-old Hinemaia, after she includes cancer in her list of illnesses. "That it could actually kill you," she replies; her nana died of cancer. While we are looking at the crosses that have been put out by the school playground to commemorate the soldiers who died in World War I, eleven-year-old Pikau tells me about her auntie who died, an auntie who had been very sick because she had a colostomy bag. Ten-year-old Chloe tells me how her church played videos of children in Pakistan who are "really sick, and if one of the boys there gets one more drink of dirty water he'll die." Cancer is memorable because it is deadly, the fates of soldiers in war are linked to a colostomy bag, and children in Pakistan must be close to dying if they are sick. In this way, sickness and death are, for Tūrama School children, entangled, as each constitutes the other.

This coupling of death and illness likely comes in part from those parents and grandparents whose death was attributed to illness, like Trystan's auntie who apparently died of pneumonia. A great weapon of structural violence is the way deaths become naturalized, ascribed to their proximate causes rather than the systemic inequalities that left those bodies vulnerable to illness in the first place. However, recent media campaigns in New Zealand that both involve children and draw on death as a motivator contribute to the meaning of death for children, as well as inadvertently targeting children with powerful, frightening messages that are meant for their parents. The One Heart Many Lives campaign, which aims to "inspire Māori and Pacific Island men to get a heart check" (PHARMAC 2017),[1] includes an advertisement aired on Māori Television showing a young girl speaking to her father about how important he is to her and to the protection of Māori *tikanga* (customs) and *taonga* (treasures). "But I'm too young to visit you in the cemetery, Dad," the girl says, sitting in tears outside the *whare nui*.[2] "See a doctor, and get your heart checked. I love you dad." This advertisement uses the tears of a grieving child to motivate fathers to have their hearts checked, but also likely impacts children who identify with the young girl and fear the loss of their fathers. Aired on the national Māori television channel, this campaign also speaks specifically to *Māori* children. Similarly, the rheumatic fever campaign, which is intended to target Māori and Pacific *parents*, in fact captures the attention of children. Many of the television and poster advertisements feature children, telling their stories with explicit links to death. "Last year, I almost died," a young boy tells the camera over a solemn piano motif and ambulance sirens. Death, as it is portrayed in these advertisements, is not the gentle, spiritual crossing over to *Te Ao Wairua* (the spiritual world) that children hear narrated at tangihanga, but one of panicked lights and sirens, alienating surgical theaters and thick scars that witness the ripping open of a body, a close evasion of a terrible fate. This death is used to connote the most extreme feelings of fear or anxiety and, in doing so, constitutes a terrifying new version of death. Importantly, although this is a framing of illness in terms of death, these advertisements feature Māori and Tongan children and, as such, directly target not only children, but specifically Māori and Pasifika children.

If death represents a powerful tool of expression for children, then portrayals of child death in the media have a particular, unrecognized potency. While children's low status and presumed passive role often renders them invisible in policy and planning, paradoxically, calls to "think about the children" are often used for the purpose of mobilizing adult action, without regard for children's interpretation of this messaging itself. The invisibility of children in society means that the Health Promotion Agency did not consider how they would view these advertisements (personal communication). However, the effect of the rheumatic fever campaign on the children of Tūrama School is very evident. Children would recite the campaign messages verbatim; ten-year-old Te Kapua, placing himself in the shoes of the boy, narrates: "My brother almost died. It started with a sore throat." Half a world away, Jean Hunleth (2017) describes a similar response among Zambian children to orphanhood discourses propagated by adults to draw attention to HIV and related illnesses. Repeating slogans they heard on the radio and in school, even children who technically already *were* orphans expressed fear of *becoming* an orphan. Children constructed a meaning of orphanhood with similar valence to the meaning of death for Tūrama School children, connoting loss of social relationships, care, and belonging.

In chapter 4, I introduced Marielle, who misunderstood her two bouts of strep throat to be "rheumatic fever," which, for her, was characterized by the experience of breathlessness, a symptom the nurse later attributed to anxious hyperventilation. Marielle's interpretation of her experience seems to have been directly shaped by the rheumatic fever television campaign, which she repeatedly references, along with her fear that she was going to die. After nearly crying from nervous excitement at the beginning of our interview, Marielle stammers as she tells me the story, her scramble for words echoing the anxiety she felt that day when she couldn't breathe.

"Well, I thought that I was gonna die becàuse it was my first time. It was my first time that I got rheumatic fever?"

I go to clarify, "You thought you were going to die—"

"—Yeah, because it was my first time."

"Because it was your first time. How come you thought you were going to die?" I wonder.

"Oh, because I couldn't breathe properly?" Marielle explains. "And because, like—like, if you have rheumatic fever, like, you have to, like—" She gasps, demonstrating. "Like, breathe like in, and then you have to, like, breathe out. It's, like, really weird. For the first time, but when you get your second, like, you'll know."

Marielle's breathlessness began when the doctor said she had rheumatic fever, and back at home she found herself processing what that meant. She knew what rheumatic fever was, because the television "said it," even though she did not know how it would feel before. Voice shaking, she tells me, "Then I was thinking, like, I was gonna be that boy?" Marielle's retelling of her strep throat experience bristles with embodied anxiety, mirroring the gasping breaths that crept upon her as she went about her day. For Marielle, the experience was "making real" the story she'd heard on the television, and, thinking that she too would be like "that boy," she stressed about taking her pills. Her sister's wedding was scheduled before the end of her antibiotics course, so to make sure she would be well for the event, Marielle took the final few days' worth all at once. When I ask her what she remembers from the television advertisement, she is vague on the details, but she remembers the death part. "It was just about how, like, when he was born his heart was, like, not—good? Then he got a surgery. Something. 'Cause his brother almost died."

This is where children's concepts of death *matter*. Adults may forget that an audience is wider than the intended target, that adult talk of death will reach children, and that children will make their own sense of what they see. Because death is such a powerful concept in children's worlds, in linking childhood and death adults inadvertently speak children's language directly to them.

For these children, rheumatic fever's representation in media campaigns discursively links illness to death, but also structures health care in terms of death management. The particular version of death that constructs narratives of rheumatic fever also drives children's practices: their attendance at the clinic, the way they take medication, even their breathing. Many children at Tūrama School expressed that they would come to the clinic to have their throats checked "in case" out of fear of death. As described in chapter 4, Dandre, afraid of the bug that will kill you, goes to the clinic so Whaea Allison can check whether he has a sore throat. His sister Jordyn associates forgetting her medication with a near-death experience and, panicking that she might die, takes her antibiotics "again and again," before she puts the sticker on her chart to confirm the medicine has been taken, and she can relax once more. Marielle conscientiously takes days' worth of pills at once to be sure she is cured by the time of her sister's wedding.

Such hypervigilance is again mirrored in Hunleth's (2017) Zambian children: fear of "orphanhood" drove children to be exceptionally vigilant in maintaining the health of their parent, while adults endeavored to remove the child from

proximity to the ill parent. Children would respond to their vulnerability by taking responsibility for the monitoring of their family members' treatment
regimes, including ensuring that the relative adhered to the treatment by bringing pills and drinking water and encouraging them to take the medicine, and
becoming quite distressed when hospitals prevented the children from monitoring treatment adherence. However, at Tūrama School, clinic nurses also identified the opposite issue, when sometimes children with badly infected throats
would avoid the clinic out of fear. Whaea Allison recounted a story of going to
visit the home of a child with repeated positive strep A results to swab the child's
siblings in an effort to stamp out the bacteria. A seven-year-old brother with a
badly infected throat refused to be swabbed because he'd seen the advertising
and didn't want to get rheumatic fever. Thus, hyper-avoidance, along with hypervigilance, could turn into a health-care strategy in the management of death. In
this way, children's concepts of death, constituted as a mode of expression in
peer cultures and shaped by the structures of childhood in socio-political context, are woven into practices and hence into the coproduction of health itself.

Conclusion

This chapter describes one account of how death appears in children's everyday,
in a context in which death is both culturally salient and demographically more
frequent. Although the previous anthropological literature dealing with child
perspectives on death has primarily considered death as an anomalous childhood event, children in many contexts have extensive contact with death, if not
through personal experience, then through the experiences of peers or representations of death in stories, media, and games. Listening for death in everyday small talk can hear how children come not only to express their sense-making
of death, but how they use death to make sense of life. As an expressive tool,
death can therefore also function as a lens for understanding the experience of
childhood.

The experience of childhood that Tūrama School children's death talk
reveals is one of embeddedness in relations of kinship and care, and of a dependency that creates precarious social positions. For children, death may invoke
not only moments of existential disconcertion, but also the social disruption that
follows the loss of a parent figure. Although, for many, close whānau ties mean
that a child who loses one or both parents will often be re-homed with other
relatives, children's dependence and lack of power leaves them structurally vulnerable to unpredictable dislocation. Death is the slipping of your feet on a
ground that has suddenly given way, with no promise of where you might land.

As a result of this structural vulnerability, their social dependency, and their
lack of power, death, then, carries special meaning for children. Children's
expressions of death, in particular a process of apprehending this unknowable

threat through a social cataloging of death events and causes, can bring into relief their experiences of vulnerability. Furthermore, the way that children use death language to express ideas about other things in their everyday discourse can also reveal the social meaning of death, and of those things. For children, the language of death comes to connote what death represents as well as its literal meaning, a shared signifier of the *scariest* experience, the *most* dangerous risks, or the *worst* illness. Yet the same structures that render children vulnerable also make them invisible to policy makers who invoke child death to persuade adults but inadvertently tap into this powerful discourse of childhood, influencing children's practices in life.

9

Conclusion

In May 2016, six months after I finished fieldwork, I visited Tūrama School again for the day. At the beginning of morning tea I was swamped with excited children who remembered me, while new faces stared with curiosity and suspicion. After five minutes they had, for the most part, run out of things to tell me and drifted back to their games.

There were many faces missing. Victor, who had the rheumatic heart condition, had not returned to Tūrama School this year, I thought perhaps because his mother Adrienne had decided to move him to a school closer to home. Teuila, who begged spinach from my sandwich and shared her antibiotics, had also not returned this year, and a teacher suggested she would now be attending a school closer to the state house her family had been allocated after the death of her father. Nga-Atawhainga and her sister Te Rerenga, Harrison, Amberlee, and Arya had all moved away. Te Kapua, Tupono, best friends Trystan and Navahn, and many others, having completed year six, had graduated to the intermediate school nearby. Some of the staff had changed as well. Deb, the nurse, was still working in the clinic, but Whaea Allison had moved on to another role and there was a new "sore throat lady" now. I was not to know it then, but within the next two years, more school staff would have moved on than would have stayed.

But I was delighted to find Cassidee, who had told me last year she thought she would be moving again, now in the year seven/eight bilingual unit. She still had her stoic poise but had paired up with Soraya, who used to be best friends with Ruby, and both girls had matching shaved undercuts, the popular hairstyle. They saw Ruby from time to time, they told me, when she came to the gate to meet her little sisters, but she didn't really speak to them. I also spent some time with Mila, who was growing into a leadership role in Mrs. Stevens's class this year. She, Hinemaia, and Dandre all proudly sported school councillor badges. Pikau, now in year eight, had grown tall and lanky, well into adolescence.

Around the time that I began writing this conclusion in 2017, a UNICEF report on child well-being in developed nations had just been released, ranking New Zealand 38 out of 40 in a measure of health and well-being across five indicators: neonatal mortality (<4 weeks), suicide rates (0–19 years), mental health symptoms (11–15 years), drunkenness (11–15 years), and teenage fertility rates (15–19 years) (UNICEF Office of Research 2017). At a rate of 15.8 per 100,000, New Zealand's youth suicide rate is the highest of any developed nation by a substantial margin. These are the issues awaiting the children of this book; as their immune systems mature and they grow out of vulnerability to rheumatic fever, they age into new demographics of risk. In the most recent report from the Ministry of Health, the rate of youth suicide in Manukau, the district health board that includes Papakura, is higher than the national average (Ministry of Health 2016). The same report shows suicide rates increasing with deprivation quintiles—a relationship strongest for the youth population, with the three most deprived quintiles experiencing four times as many suicides as the least deprived. Māori and Pasifika young men between fifteen and twenty-five are the two most at-risk groups, followed by Māori women and European men in the same age bracket. The highest rates of hospitalizations for intentional self-harm were recorded for young Māori and Pākehā women in the fifteen-to-twenty-four age group living in neighborhoods of high deprivation (Ministry of Health 2016). It seems that the environments many of our young people are maturing in are not even close to providing the resources for thriving.

In conservation science, sentinel species are organisms that are particularly sensitive or manifest early responses to environmental change and thus are used as bio-monitors, signaling early warnings of contaminants or declining ecological systems. Across time and space, different indicators may emerge within particular sectors of society that represent "sentinel diseases": a canary in the coal mine for inequitable conditions, or a warning sign of deeper faults in housing and socioeconomic circumstances that will also manifest in a broad range of other health issues. Such indicators—diabetes; cardiovascular disease; meningococcal B; low birth weight; and, currently in New Zealand, rheumatic fever— may not be the earliest signs of deteriorating environments, but their measurability and reliable connection to environmental circumstances mean they can function as proxies for material inequities, racism, or spiritual dislocation (Walters, Mohammed, Evans-Campbell, et al. 2011).

Yet because treating the canary with antibiotics can show quantifiable effects, attempted treatment of isolated diseases through "targeted" approaches to public health may be preferred not only for financial reasons, but also to allow governments to demonstrate progress to those to whom they are accountable.

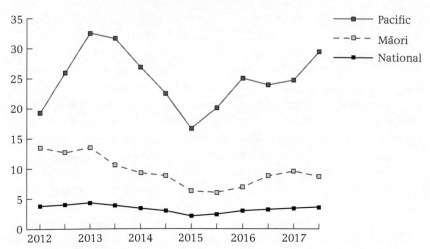

FIGURE 10 Rheumatic fever rates in New Zealand from 2012 to 2018. Data source: Ministry of Health, 2018.

As a Better Public Services (BPS) target of the National Party government, the goal of the Rheumatic Fever Prevention Programme was to cut rheumatic fever admissions by two-thirds by June 2017. In the year leading up to July 1, 2017, this program saw only a 15 percent reduction in rheumatic fever cases overall—in real terms, from 177 cases in 2012, to 160 in 2017 (Ministry of Health 2017). The rate in the Counties Manukau district, where Tūrama School is located, dropped from 14.6 to 10.2 cases per 100,000, and this district retained the highest rate nationally by a large margin (compared with the 2017 national average rate of 3.4 per 100,000). Nationwide statistics show a steady decline for Māori rates over the period of the program, but these high Auckland rates particularly reflect the Pasifika statistics, which, after dipping in 2014–2015, spiked again in late 2015, and in 2016 reached the same levels as in 2012 (Figure 10). For all the targeted interventions, Pasifika peoples have seen little change.

The 15 percent decrease nationwide falls well below the targeted reduction of 67 percent, but was enough for the government to claim success and commit funding for another five years to rheumatic fever prevention. The problem here, of course, is that while children have been fortified with antibiotics, the conditions that created the epidemic remain in place. Indeed, the statistics published in December 2018 show that rheumatic fever rates are even higher than 2017, at a rate of 3.6 per 100,000 nationally, and 14.7 per 100,000 for the Counties-Manukau district (Ministry of Health, 2018). Yet scaling back the interventions would leave children at risk again, and removal of the school clinics would leave a cohort of children, attuned to sore throat risk and conditioned to seek treatment, with no place to go.

New Directions in Child Policy

Yet the political milieu that seemed so entrenched and stagnant just a few months ago now anticipates a potentially significant new direction. An unexpected change of government in late 2017 through a coalition agreement has seen a rapid reprioritizing, at least in rhetoric, of child poverty issues in Aotearoa. An early move of the new, left-leaning government has been to scrap the BPS targets of which reducing rheumatic fever rates represented one (unmet) target. Instead of targeting streptococcus infections, the government has announced it will be focusing on systemic change—addressing the overcrowding and child poverty that underlie rheumatic fever rates (New Zealand Government 2018). Although exactly what this will look like remains unclear, it appears that the New Zealand government's approach of medicating the canary may be shifting toward changing the coal mine.

Meanwhile, the outgoing National Party, which until the 2017 election disputed both the number of children in poverty and the measurability of child poverty (Moir 2016), criticized the new Labour Party government's child poverty reduction proposals as under-ambitious, and, now in opposition after nine years in power, has signaled that it will support the government's proposed legislation only if amendments are made to reintroduce BPS targets and "hold the public service accountable" (New Zealand National Party 2018). Hon. Paula Bennett, who as Minister of Social Development rejected legislation to provide children in poverty with free lunch on the grounds of "parental responsibility" (see chapter 5), now states her expectation as the National Party Spokesperson for Children that the government would "address the drivers of social dysfunction" and use "social investment models" so that families and communities get the resources they need. Children are therefore very much implicated in current contestations for political power, although it remains to be seen whether any material change will result for the incoming cohorts of Tūrama School children. Nevertheless, while Aotearoa still trails countries such as Sweden for child-centered policy (D'Souza 2017) there appears to be fresh reconsideration of the role the state plays—whether through action or inaction—in shaping children's health and welfare.

Without understating the significant impact of the state and society on children's health, in this book the case of rheumatic fever prevention has been the entry point for a different set of questions, this time about the role children themselves play in the production of their health. Children may be increasingly the focus of policy change, but still missing is a view of children as social actors, whose experiences, understandings, interpretations, and practices matter and can powerfully mediate the success or failure of policy interventions. Instead, the trend in New Zealand, as well as internationally, has been toward what scholars describe as an "elevation" of children within neoliberal policy, with the purpose of targeting "vulnerable" children for intervention within a social-investment paradigm concerned with reducing future costs to the state (Elizabeth and Larner 2009; Keddell 2018; O'Brien 2016). The rheumatic fever prevention program is an archetypal example here, along with recent changes to child protection policy that channel resources into identifying and policing at-risk families rather than providing support or addressing chronic entrenched poverty, material deprivation, and mental health issues (Cleland 2016; Keddell 2018).

This, therefore, is "child-focused" policy, but it is rarely child-centered, in that the agenda is designed for the benefit of the taxpayer rather than for the child; legislation that punishes families for poverty is not particularly helpful for children, and impacts on children are not considered from their perspectives. Other examples of this tendency to overlook the importance of children's views can also be seen in recent changes to family law that eliminated the rights of children to have a lawyer representing their views in family court unless there are concerns for the child's safety; in the Adoption Act 1955, which has no requirement for the court to hear from the child (Cleland 2013); and in the rebranding of Child, Youth and Family Services to the stigmatizing and controversial "Ministry for Vulnerable Children" (although another early move of the incoming government was to remove the word "vulnerable" from this name).

Fitzmaurice (2017) notes that Aotearoa lacks the *participation ecosystem*—the participatory culture, infrastructure, understanding, and research—needed to allow children's perspectives to shape institutions, practices, and services in ways that are useful and meaningful for children. When children's perspectives are included, such as in the recent consultative processes for the reformed child protection services (Fitzmaurice 2017), these processes still tend to remain adult-centric, transplanting children into adult political arenas (Lansdown 2010) and with an emphasis on voice, meaning the verbal sharing of children's experiences, views, and opinions, which privileges the views of older and more articulate children. While children can certainly express rich and valuable perspectives, as many did in the present study, a child-centered approach to policy must also hear children's many nonverbal expressions and situate these in the ecological, relational, cultural, and institutional contexts within which these expressions have been produced. Doing so requires knowing children's lives—embodied, negotiated, and embedded in relationships—beyond what children might name in an interview in a strange place with strange adults. The ethnographic mode of "being there" (Borneman and Hammoudi 2009) is particularly useful for understanding the perspectives of children who may be less practiced at verbal articulation but who can nonetheless express their experiences through multiple other embodied or relational modes. Such an understanding of children's lives would better allow the systematic and reflexive suspension of adult-centric lenses and dominant social conceptions of children so that processes and policies can instead be seen from the child's-eye view. Such an understanding also allows consideration of potential effects of policy decisions on children's practices, whether that is the way a stigmatizing ministry name may affect children's peer relationships or the way a rheumatic fever campaign may create hypervigilant health practices.

How Do Children Participate in the Coproduction of Their Health?

How, then, should we conceptualize children's contributions to their health in the context of their lives? While researchers embrace questions of how children *experience* health and illness, children's interpretations and practices rarely figure into analyses of the *production* of child health. In New Zealand, such analyses take the form of mainly longitudinal quantitative studies (Fergusson, Boden, and Horwood 2015; Savila, Sundborn, Hirao, et al. 2011; Morton, Atatoa Carr, Grant, et al. 2013; Silva 1990), in which, perhaps, children are presumed to be passive, or their activities are disregarded as inconsequential, or their social action is assumed to be the product of their environment and what adults are doing. Some of the reticence to seriously consider children's practices may stem from an idea that children *ought not* be consequential players in their health, that children's health should be produced by adults, or at the very most that children's role should be learning to take care of themselves as they are taught at home and school. To focus on children's contributions to their health status risks making them responsible for their well-being or shifts attention from the many ways that their health is influenced by people and social forces with far greater power. Yet how would our understanding of child health change if we were to include a view of children's interpretive practices as part of the analysis?

I have argued throughout this book that such a view of children's activities would reveal that children's practices, generated through collective peer cultures and in relation to wider social structures, have significant potential to structure their health. I have shown how children's interpretive practices can shape their nutritional status, use of pharmaceuticals, engagements with health care, allostatic adjustments of the body's internal milieu, social support, and exposure to risk. These practices can also influence the success or failure of policy or institutional interventions intended to facilitate children's well-being. These are not particularly new findings. Similar sorts of practices can be found throughout the existing interpretive literature on children's health and illness: how children employ imaginative strategies to cope with chronic illness (Clark 2003); how children interpret their bodies in culturally specific ways and consequently may under- or over-report symptoms (Christensen 1999); how children within peer cultures stigmatize some forms of illness (runny noses, eczema) (James 1993); how children attempt to stay in proximity to and care for an ill parent (Hunleth 2017). There are clear implications of these practices for children's own health;

we might anticipate they mediate treatment adherence or efficacy, timing or accuracy of diagnosis, social support and well-being, or exposure to pathogens. These are not inconsequential effects, but in this literature the conversation is not about how these activities help to *make* child health.

How, then, can children's practices be integrated into conversations about the production of child health? How can we represent children's agency in analyses of rheumatic fever, obesity, or depression without implying children are responsible for their health status, making their behaviors into targets of intervention, or detracting attention from structural inequities and injustices? One solution has been offered by the social ecology models of childhood resilience (Panter-Brick, Theron, Liebenberg, et al. 2015; Ungar 2011; Ungar, Ghazinour, and Richter 2013), discussed in chapter 7, which attempt to include children as social actors who negotiate their own well-being in relation to environments that constrain or open up resources to facilitate young people's practices. This sets up a way of giving attention to children's practices as strategic choices made from a limited number of available options, and, in view of children's circumstances, practices that may seem counterproductive from adult perspectives can be understood as accommodations that balance costs and benefits across different domains in resource-poor or challenging contexts. A view of what children do is valued here for understanding how to improve environments and resources in ways that will give children better options or mitigate the costs of what children do.

Working from psychology and social work fields (although also picked up in the large-scale anthropological work of Catherine Panter-Brick [e.g., Panter-Brick, Theron, Liebenberg, et al. 2015]) the social ecology model tends to take an individualized and unidirectional view of children responding to the conditions of their environment. What the ethnographic data from Tūrama School show, however, is the way that children's practices are deeply interconnected and, as such, work to help create the environments that constrain and open up opportunities and resources. Children like Ruby work within peer ecologies to create friendship groups that stabilize an unstable world but, at the same time, Ruby's practices create new vulnerabilities for the children she excludes. Boys like Harrison, who employ aggression to maintain their social safety, create unsafe environments for their targets. Children technically have access to spare lunches, but the social meanings they collectively ascribe to these mean that this form of resource is constrained by social costs, while other forms of provisions, like the milk, are woven into collective and *enabling* social rituals. This dialectic, in which children collectively co-construct the structures that guide their action, is not quite captured in existing models.

I have therefore argued that a coproduction framework offers another way for us to make room for children's agency by positioning children as working in dialectical relationship with adults, the body, and wider social structures including the state, the institution, cultural ideologies, and the economy. Coproduction, as I have used the term—the way that children, society, and the body make one another—recognizes that children do not simply internalize but also creatively *produce* culture (Corsaro 1992). Yet these cultural meanings and practices, on the one hand, are structured by experiences of the body and wider social systems, and on the other, mediate the relationships between wider social systems and the body; they are coproducing and coproduced. Thus, Tūrama School children construct understandings of sore throat at the interface between their experience of the body incarnate and a political agenda that targets sore throats within health-care systems (chapter 4), and they interpret provisions as acceptable or stigmatized care through their own notions of intergenerational roles and responsibilities (chapter 5). From their experience of structural vulnerability, children make meanings of death in terms of illness and threat to the social (chapter 8). Meanwhile, these cultural meanings themselves form structuring social systems that guide children's practices and become embodied as a particular form of habitus (Bourdieu 1984), directly shaping their health. Peer cultures create systems that constrain food resources or open up access to health care, which then structure how bodily signals of hunger, cold, or sore throat are experienced, interpreted, and responded to (chapter 6). Children's understandings of social relations, responsibility for care, illness, medicine, and their own bodily sensations influence how they engage with health care, patterns of nutrition, or practices of using pharmaceuticals (chapters 4–5). Children strategically employ practices of resilience to enable coping in one domain of health (e.g., peer society), but these may come at a cost in another (e.g., risk of physical injury) (chapter 7). Through these processes children translate their politically and economically structured experiences of the world and of their body into local social meanings and practices, which in turn help to shape future action and future bodies. Children's health activities— building relationships, caring for their body, eating and drinking, taking medicine, engaging in risk—are all coproductions authored by society, families, institutions, and children themselves. Children are not solely the ones responsible for their health here, but institutions and policy makers are made responsible for considering how children will understand and respond to the conditions of their childhood and for taking children's meanings and practices into account in designing or evaluating policy or social services.

Viewing children's health as a coproduction enables us to value and give attention to children's efforts to manage their own lives and support the health of others. In practice, as well, acknowledging the role children play within these dynamics allows us to better predict the effectiveness of policy decisions or, better still, to design interventions and services that align with and support children's ideas and goals. Such an approach might ask, What would school lunches look like if created with a view of how food functions within children's social relations? How would rheumatic fever policy change if we began by asking what a sore throat means to children? What if child protection began not with how we can identify, monitor, and police "at-risk" families, but how we can support and preserve those aspects of families that children value and are trying to make for themselves? There may be a near-consensus that poverty is bad for children but, when viewed through children's eyes, some responses to child poverty are also bad for children. From children's perspectives, material resources may matter less than the effects those resources have on family relations, time, and affective care. What kinds of resources, delivered in what way, would make the biggest difference to what children need and value?

A coproduction framework also allows us to better understand how the systems that generate health inequalities operate through childhood experience and how society discursively and structurally positions children and influences their activities. When viewed as coproductions, children's perspectives and practices tell us something about the way society is structured to create ethnic, economic, or generational vulnerabilities and how these are experienced. The way children use the language of death in association with illness speaks to the precariousness with which they view their lives, and how health inequities destabilize children's social relationships and sharpen their perceptions of risk. A coproduction framework may also be applied outside of health, as an analytical tool that moves beyond socialization or internalization for understanding how children contribute to other aspects of their childhoods.

Finally, viewing children's activities as a coproduction also means considering the ways that children contribute to their coproduction partners: how children help to support adult health, how children modify institutions, how children influence society. Children's lack of social or political power can sometimes be mistaken for a lack of effect; however, children shape economies as consumers (Buckingham 2011) as well as laborers (Kramer 2005; Nag, White, Peet, et al. 1978), act as language brokers for immigrant parents (Orellana 2009), and co-construct learning exchanges with grandparents (Kenner, Ruby, Jessel, et al. 2007). Jean Hunleth's (2017) work on children's roles in caring for parents with tuberculosis—what could be termed the coproduction of family health—argues for the importance of not limiting consideration of children to "children's issues" or only those activists, researchers, and policy makers concerned with children. For Hunleth, the invisibility of children from the perspectives of health professionals caring for adults, and attempts to remove children from adult tuberculosis sufferers, were in themselves harmful to children. Likewise, at Tūrama School, the invisibility of children to rheumatic fever campaign designers created anxious children. As illustrated by Mila's story in chapter 7, the activities and positions of children and adults are intertwined, so just as parents fret over taking their child with a sore throat to the doctor, children will worry about a parent who frets. Social discourse therefore cannot speak of parents without speaking to children, and vice versa. A coproduction framework can remind us to look for children's influences, as well as how they are impacted, in studies of adults or society more broadly.

This book has been about elevating the unseen and underestimated practices of childhood in the social theory of health and of society more broadly. I have also spoken to how we should consider childhood in *practice*: of grounding policy in understandings of children's experiences and activities as they are lived in situ. Most important for me, this book has been about listening to and hearing from a group of children who feature regularly in public discourse as statistics and stereotypes, but whose stories as *people* are rarely heard. The word "tūrama" means light, and I named Tūrama School for the shining little humans I saw every day. Many of these children suffer greatly from the effects of structural violence, but their lives are also about helping friends and joking with teachers, sneaking lollies to share, loving their parents and grandparents, taking pride in their mathematics and soccer and art, caring, grieving, singing, fighting, resisting, and trying. These are the children in child health, and they are the most bright and brilliant humans I have known.

Appendix

Drawing Child Ethnography

The illustrations of this book reflect the important role that visual modes of expression—from both myself and my participants—played throughout my fieldwork at Tūrama School. Although I did not set out to produce visual ethnography, I had always intended to collect children's artwork as data, and many times over I invited children to draw, suggesting, as a prompt, that they might draw either something they enjoyed at school or a time when things were tough. From this process, children like Cassidee (chapter 8) gifted me with the illustrations which first helped me to recognize just how unstable these children's worlds were and how much grief they carried around the disruption of their relationships. This is not something I often heard from them in direct conversation, and these drawings opened up new ways of understanding how children experienced their world. Yet while drawing has a long history as a methodological tool in research with children (see Bluebond-Langner 1978; Hunleth 2011), it is less common for *researchers* to engage in drawing practices; the drawing is for children, while researchers tend get on with the "real" business of interviewing or taking notes.

I had not, therefore, considered how my own artistic practices might also contribute to the production of this research. Although I hold a graduate degree in fine arts, I had entered anthropology for the science of understanding people and held a very conventional focus on translating my data into written form. Yet almost as soon as I began working with children, I also began drawing, painting, or taking photographs, artistic practices that are woven into the fabric of school and home life. I illustrated stories and drew diagrams of volcanoes in my exercise book, and taught children to make clay masks and expressionist paintings in an art class. I photographed school trips and costume days, and guided children in a photography project of their own. I painted banners for school sports days and face-painted for the school fair. These practices gave me ways of participating *with* children in their worlds, providing me with a role and a means to contribute, and facilitating social interactions, as Ramos (2004, 137) has also described, "part of the anthropological process of tentatively bringing together observer and observed." I quickly became aware that I gained cultural capital from my drawing skills, which children admire and value. Drawing allowed me to build connections with children who were also artistically inclined; boys who would normally ignore or avoid me would talk to me about my drawing and show me theirs. Nine-year-old Teuila, a prolific artist herself, took an interest in my face-paints and so I gave her a lesson one lunchtime and bought her a set of paints and brushes at the end of the year.

Meanwhile, I drew alongside children in interviews, which helped children feel more comfortable and open talking to me, as not all my attention was focused on them and the shared activity was conducive to rapport. Yet with all this focus on the drawing process as a relational tool, and on children's draw-ings as ethnographic stories, it did not occur to me until quite late that my own drawings were more than a means to the "real" data but could be valuable eth-nographic representations in and of themselves. By this stage, I had already given many of my drawings away to the children in exchange for theirs.

My drawing-as-data emerged toward the end of my fieldwork as I worked alongside the children to produce an ethnography for them—a picture book that I intended as a way of reporting back to my child participants and acknowledg-ing what I had found. During our interview, Teuila the artist and I found our-selves drawing each other—she drawing me drawing her—and the composite I made of these drawings formed the opening spread of the picture book. As I was drawing so much anyway, it started to make sense to include some of my draw-ings with theirs, and I also started producing more finished drawings of the children and aspects of school life, several of which now feature in this book. Although *children's* drawings have long been used in research, I began to recog-nize, as have others, that *ethnographer* drawings have advantages beyond facili-tating relationships.

If the goal of ethnography is to create a sense of "being there," then a bur-geoning literature on visual anthropology demonstrates the capacity of artistic and sensory modes of data collection to enrich the re-creating of fieldwork experiences. Scholars like Sarah Pink (2013) note that visual representations can allow us to access an embodied way of understanding how participants and eth-nographers feel, see, and experience the world they are living in or studying. Drawing, in particular, offers ways of representing aspects of people's experi-ences that cannot be recounted verbally or photographically. In my case, the need to protect participant confidentiality means that I have hundreds of beau-tiful photographs that I can never use. But I can *draw* them.

Drawing is not just a second-rate alternative to photography, however. Michael Taussig (2011, 13) writes that "drawing intervenes in the reckoning of reality in ways that writing and photography do not." I understand this to mean that drawing isn't trying to be reality or a proxy for truth. Drawing is, very honestly, a *representing*. It is a reconstructing of a moment through the subjective perspective of the drawer; it is recomposing an environment, recorporealizing actors into their bodily form and repositioning them in space. Drawing is to show the viewer the impression I have in my mind's eye, not just the view of my physical eye. A layer of interpretation is added: the sharpness and fuzziness of memory, of who is central and who is peripheral, of how a body and its environment *felt* more than exactly what it looked like. Drawing captures the embodied experience of the drawer, partly because the process of drawing is an embodied and sensory form of labor, coordinating hand, eye, memory toward a material thing of which every mark says, "This is how I saw, this is what I want to express." Drawings emerge through a period of labor, of sketching, adjusting, erasing, refining, that mirrors the writing process, often leaving the vestiges of that editing process as indents on the paper. The manufacture is part of the data.

Particular to this research about children's embodied practices, through drawings I found I could attend to the body in ways limited in written description alone. Indeed, my representations of what I experienced and saw in the field have in common a close attention to the way children held and used their bodies, how bodies expressed affection and vulnerability and power, and how bodies existed in space and in relation to one another—and in relation to me. Fieldwork at Tūrama School was so primordially *physical*, from the children snuggling into my side from the very first day, to the sticky sourness of sweat-slicked limbs in a stifling classroom after a lunchtime of soccer, to the tense freeze that swept a class when an authority figure slammed a desk. Life at Tūrama School felt so much more physical than my actual, adult life, in which boundaries between bodies are so constantly and conscientiously policed. It is this embodiedness that I have tried to capture, if not in the text, then in the illustrations in this book, whether they are of those bodies twisting around poles and railings, huddling to keep warm, or stoically enduring a throat swab.

This was also the etic view I brought to the picture book, alongside children's emic perspectives as rendered in colored pens. In this picture book, drawing also offered an avenue for coproducing research, although I acknowledge children's pictures were still interpreted and edited through my adult gaze. The final product stands alone as a visual ethnography for a child audience, with copies printed for every child who had contributed a drawing or participated in an interview, for each classroom, and for the school library, as well as viewable online. Drawing therefore functioned first to create relationships and then lastly to close and memorialize them. However, the visual ethnography children seemed to value most of all was not the one they had coproduced, but the moments captured in the photographs I had taken. Between my own photography and children commandeering my phone for "selfies," I had accumulated a large bank of photographs, and I printed the nicest portraits for the children to keep as a goodbye gift. Because children have little access to equipment, money, or transport to have their own photographs taken and printed, these snapshots, which, at a few cents each, cost me substantially less to print than the books, were seized, compared, and exclaimed over. While a drawing can convey a lot, it was in the photographs that children really saw themselves. The drawings, then, are for the rest of the world, to show you what we saw.

ACKNOWLEDGMENTS

As the outcome of years of doctoral research, this book is very much a coproduction, and I owe the deepest gratitude to the many contributors who helped to bring the story of Tūrama School to life.

I was fortunate to have the opportunity to develop this research and subsequent book under the rigorous supervision of Susanna Trnka and Judith Littleton. Thank you for challenging me when you knew I could be challenged, while giving me the space to write about what I loved. Their efforts were supplemented by many wonderful people at the University of Auckland who, over the years, offered comments on drafts, care and encouragement, and general kicks in the right direction. For all of your contributions to this process, I especially thank Phyllis Herda, Christine Dureau, Julie Park, Cris Shore, Bruce Floyd, Sally Raudon, Anneka Anderson, and all members of the Social Anthropology Thesis Writer's Group and Biological Anthropology Writer's Group. This research was generously supported by a University of Auckland Doctoral Scholarship. I would like to thank Brian Joyce at Papakura marae for sharing your experiences of your community, and further afield, many thanks to Helen Lee and Jean Hunleth for your ongoing encouragement and suggestions.

I was fortunate to have the support of many compassionate and generous friends and mentors who formed a valuable and stable support network throughout the production and aftermath of this research: among others, Ash Mathur, Mythily Meher, Jasmine Taylor, Shyla Kelly, Val Leveson, Avi Clark, Rhyll Stafford, and Shanthi Ameratunga. A special ngā mihi nui to my dear friend Nga-Atawhainga Manukau, who gifted me many of the names used as pseudonyms in this book, including those of her three children: Pikau, Ngapaea, and Tupono.

Thank you to my mother, Jane Spray, for your interest and for sharing your teacher experiences as points of comparison. Thank you to my partner, Simon Keeling, along with the greater Keeling whānau, for accepting me and my many moments of grumpy introversion with love and understanding over the past few years.

The greatest contributors I cannot name here because my ethical obligations mean I must keep you anonymous. Thank you to "Tūrama School" for hosting me for my fieldwork: to the principal and board of trustees, staff, and families. Thank you to the parents who trusted me to talk to your babies, and even more to the parents who trusted me to talk to you. The biggest thanks must go to my child participants, who shared your games, your experiences, your drawings, and your friendship. I am honoured to be kaitiaki of your kōrero.

GLOSSARY

Some Māori words are not easily translatable into English. So as not to disrupt sentence clarity, some words requiring more detailed explanations are footnoted. Māori translations are referenced from the *Te Aka Māori-English Dictionary* (Moorfield 2011).

Where children have anglicized Māori words, for example by pluralizing words by adding "s," I have represented the hybridized word as they have used it in context.

All words are Māori unless specified otherwise.

aiga (Samoan). wider family

Aotearoa. New Zealand

hapū. sub-tribe/clan

hui. meeting

iwi. tribe

kai. food, eating

kainga (Tongan). extended family

kapa haka. Māori cultural performance

kaumātua. elder

marae. a central gathering place for Māori, technically meaning the courtyard in from of the whare nui (main meeting house) but often referring to the key buildings of the complex

Pākehā. New Zealander of European ancestry (see chapter 2 for further discussion)

pōhara. poor, impoverished

poi. light balls on the end of strings that are rhythmically swung to accompany waiata

tangata whenua. indigenous people of a land

tangihanga, tangi. Māori funeral, rites for the dead, weeping

taonga. treasure

Te Ao Māori. the Māori world

Te Ao Wairua. the spiritual world

Te Reo. the (Māori) language

tikanga. correct procedure, custom

tūrama. light, to give light to, illuminate

waiata. song, to sing

wairua. spirit, soul

whaea. mother or aunty

whakapapa. genealogy, lineage, descent

whānau. extended family, family group (see note 8 of chapter 1 for further detail)

whāngai. adopted (usually informally) child

whare nui. meeting house, main building of a marae, where guests are accommodated and meetings held

NOTES

CHAPTER 1   INTRODUCTION

1. Names of all children, parents, school staff, the school itself, and other local schools have been changed to pseudonyms so as to protect the confidentiality of participants.

2. Children's speech from interviews, transcribed verbatim, has been lightly edited for clarity. I have not altered their grammar. Interactions outside of formal interviews were not recorded and so appear as reconstructions.

3. "Aotearoa," commonly translated as "land of the long white cloud," is the Māori name for New Zealand, and its use is widespread in New Zealand.

4. "Pasifika" is a pan-ethnic term used in New Zealand to describe the diverse collective of people with genealogical connections to the Pacific Islands, including Samoa, Tonga, Cook Islands, Niue, Tuvalu, and Tokelau.

5. State housing is low-cost rental housing owned and managed by the government.

6. The DHB is the governing body responsible for funding and providing health care to the local region.

7. In July 2017, as part of a suite of changes, the name of this landmark legislation was changed to the Oranga Tamariki Act 1989 and the Children's and Young People's Well-Being Act 1989.

8. Though primary school usually ends after year six, children in the bilingual classes may continue up to year eight.

9. Although sometimes used by Westerners as a broad equivalent for the English word "family," "whānau" and Pacific equivalents designate a much broader group and deeper emotional and tribal allegiance (Ritchie and Ritchie 1979). In modern New Zealand, the inclusive valence of "whānau" has also become commonly used to refer to close-knit communities of people who are not relatives, such as work teams or community groups, indicating a relationship that is "like" a family. "Whānau" can also be used refer to Māori communities more broadly (and can include Pasifika).

10. Bourdieu (1984) similarly describes an embodiment of gender in terms of tastes and bodily expressions (190–192).

CHAPTER 2   THE WORLD OF TŪRAMA SCHOOL

1. Countdown is a local supermarket chain.

2. "Pākehā" is a Māori word that has entered mainstream New Zealand English and generally refers to a New Zealander of European ancestry. Although in widespread use,

the term is contested; it featured in the 1996 census alongside New Zealand European, the official census category, but was subsequently removed, to ongoing controversy as many white New Zealanders prefer to identify as Pākehā. Use of the term is a relatively recent development, which King (1985) argues emerged in response to the Māori renaissance of the 1970s and 1980s, and implies European ancestry but indexes relationship to country as one of the "founding peoples" of the new nation state and relationship to Māori as the other.

3. Percentages are based on Education Review Office report. Many children at Tūrama School had both Māori and Pacific ancestry (or Māori and Pākehā) but were designated as Māori.

4. Following numerous reports of present and historical mismanagement leading to abuse of children under CYF care, the agency was replaced by the controversial Ministry for Vulnerable Children (also known as Tamariki Ora) in 2017. Children, teachers, and parents still commonly refer to the agency as "CYFs."

5. Kapa haka is a Māori cultural performance.

6. A marae is a central gathering place for Māori.

7. Further to long-standing criticisms of mistreatment of children under CYF's care, the rebranded Oranga Tamariki again came under public scrutiny in 2019 after a high-profile attempt to uplift a Māori newborn. Protesters, including academics and the Children's Commissioner, argued the disproportionate number of Māori children uplifted (and subsequently abused in care) reflects institutional racism and colonialism and represents a structural violence which continues to disrupt connections to whānau, whakapapa, and culture, perpetuating traumas and spiritual alienation for Māori.

CHAPTER 3   NEGOTIATING GENERATIONAL DIFFERENCES
IN ETHICAL RESEARCH

1. Various limitations to accessing and building relationships with my participants were posed by differences in ethnic and cultural background; class; and, for half the participants, gender. However, it was the generational differences—specifically the intersection of these other identity categories with generational differences—that created relational tensions in the field. While other teacher aides were from the local Māori community and parents of children at the school, I was ethnically marked as aligning with the Pākehā senior teachers and management.

2. Both sets of cultural values are also embedded in the principles of ethical guidelines: confidentiality versus protection.

CHAPTER 4   COPRODUCING HEALTH AT THE SCHOOL CLINIC

1. An earlier version of this chapter was published as Julie Spray (2018), "The Value of Anthropology in Child Health Policy," *Anthropology in Action* 25 (1): 29–40.

2. "Whaea" translates to "mother" or "aunty" and is used as an honorific indicating relative status of the speaker to the addressed—a close equivalent to "Mrs." or "Ms." The children addressed some teachers and staff with "Whaea" or the male equivalent "Matua," and others with the English honorific, depending on the person's preference.

CHAPTER 5   RESPONSIBILIZING CARE

1. "Scabbing" refers to the practice of asking or begging for food (or money) and is seen as shameful or annoying.

2. This strategy did not, however, relieve the discomfort of doing fieldwork amid such inequality in my home country. I got to eat my lunch, but I did not feel good about it.

3. As meager as this sounds, the school nurses, weighing children with sore throats to determine their antibiotic dosage, noticed that children's weights tended to be lower after the school holidays. The nurses suggested that the eating routines built into the school day ensured children were typically eating more at school than they would at home.

4. Children's dislike of peanut butter could well be the result of its almost invariable presence in spare lunches.

5. The program is not officially classified as medical "screening"—a label that brings with it particular ethical standards as a result of the increased anxiety screening produces—because only children who are identified as showing symptoms are checked. I would argue that class checks and teacher questioning to identify symptoms constitute screening—if not by medical definitions, then at least in effect.

CHAPTER 6   EMBODYING INEQUALITY

1. Emily Martin asks similar questions of how medical perspectives and work structures shape women's experiences of menstruation (1999, 1988).

2. Similar processes may occur in domestic spaces, such as toileting before bed, but to a lesser degree than at school, and these routines may be more tailored to the needs of individual children at home.

3. Poi are light balls on the end of strings that are rhythmically swung to accompany waiata.

4. Teacher responses also varied within Tūrama School and at different times, from a blind eye to wry resignation and sarcasm—"Sit here and eat your highly nutritious morning teas"—to the period of intense monitoring carried out over several weeks by Mrs. Charles, described in chapter 5.

5. This came in other variations—"I don't eat lunch," "I don't like to eat at school"—but was a very common refrain.

6. "Ow" is a vernacular form, loosely meaning "you," associated with Polynesian youth and popularized by the catchphrase "not even ow" from the 2004–2009 animated series *bro'Town*.

CHAPTER 7   PRACTICING RESILIENCE

1. This may also be a much more culturally relevant model of resilience as it moves away from a premise of Western individualism.

2. Parallels between the subjectivities of children and women in this way have been noted by Berry Mayall (1994).

3. Layne, Warren, Watson, and Shalev (2007) note that there are as many as eight different definitions of resilience in the trauma literature alone.

4. At Tūrama School, mixed year-group classes and a high prevalence of overweight or obesity may have mitigated this effect as the range of shapes and sizes expanded the

range of "normal" within the cohort, though those at either end of the wide spectrum could still be rendered more vulnerable.

5. The importance of physical competence to children was demonstrated to me every time I entered the playground; I would be mobbed by children calling, "Julie, watch me!" They would rip my gaze away from one another, competing for my attention and acknowledgment as they performed an array of jumping, twirling, balancing, and swinging skills. Sometimes they would demand that I try performing the trick and would be politely satisfied when I gave in and demonstrated my inadequacy.

6. This behavior has also been known over the years as self-injury, self-mutilation, deliberate self-harm, nonsuicidal self-injury (NSSI), and parasuicide.

7. The addition, still controversial, was mainly to distinguish the behavior from attempted suicide and from borderline personality disorder, the only other disorder for which NSSI was a criterion (Wilkinson and Goodyer 2011). The diagnostic criteria include engaging in the self-injury on five or more days in the past year, without suicidal intent, and motivated by seeking relief from a negative state, resolving an interpersonal difficulty, or inducing a positive state, excluding "socially sanctioned" behaviors (so as not to catch so-called normative practices such as tattooing, body piercing, or drinking alcohol in the wrong net). Given that many of the criteria are based on individual motivations, it is difficult to assess how many of the girls I worked with would have met the diagnosis, but most of these ten- and eleven-year-old girls likely did.

8. As this was at the very end of the school year, I was not aware of whether the effect of this disciplining was to halt the practice entirely or simply drive it into secrecy. (I, of course, would also no longer be allowed in on the secret, since I had made it clear that I was obligated to let someone know.)

CHAPTER 8   TALKING WITH DEATH

1. The campaign was led by PHARMAC (New Zealand's pharmaceutical management agency) from 2008 to 2013 and is now held within local communities.

2. The whare nui is the main building of a marae, where guests are accommodated and *hui* (meetings) are held.

REFERENCES

Adler, Patricia A., and Peter Adler. 1987. *Membership Roles in Field Research*. Newbury Park, CA: Sage.

———. 2011. *The Tender Cut: Inside the Hidden World of Self-Injury*. New York: New York University Press.

Alanen, Leena. 2001. "Explorations in Generational Analysis." In *Conceptualizing Child-Adult Relations*, ed. Leena Alanen and Berry Mayall, 11–22. New York: Routledge Falmer.

Alanen, Leena, E. Brooker, and Berry Mayall, eds. 2015. *Childhood with Bourdieu*. London: Palgrave McMillan.

American Psychiatric Association, ed. 2013. *Diagnostic and Statistical Manual of Mental Disorders, Fifth Edition*. Arlington, VA: American Psychiatric Association.

Amore, Kate. 2016. "Severe Housing Deprivation in Aotearoa/New Zealand: 2001–2013." Wellington: He Kainga Oranga/Housing & Health Research Programme, University of Otago.

Andersen, Louise Buhl. 2012. "Children's Caregiving of HIV-Infected Parents Accessing Treatment in Western Kenya: Challenges and Coping Strategies." *African Journal of AIDS Research* 11 (3): 203–213.

Anderson, N. E., D. F. Gorman, and D. R. Lines. 1977. "The Nutritional Status of Auckland Children." *New Zealand Medical Journal* 85 (580): 49–52.

Anderson, Philippa, Julian King, Michelle Moss, Phil Light, Tracy McKee, Elizabeth Farrell, Joanna Stewart, and Diana R. Lennon. 2016. "Nurse-Led School-Based Clinics for Rheumatic Fever Prevention and Skin Infection Management: Evaluation of Mana Kidz Programme in Counties Manukau." *New Zealand Medical Journal* 129 (1428): 36–45.

André, Géraldine, and Mathieu Hilgers. 2015. "Childhood in Africa between Local Powers and Global Hierachies." In *Childhood with Bourdieu*, ed. Leena Alanen, E. Brooker, and Berry Mayall, 102–141. London: Palgrave Macmillan.

Andresen, Sabine. 2014. "Childhood Vulnerability: Systematic, Structural, and Individual Dimensions." *Child Indicators Research* 7 (4): 699–713. Available from https://doi.org/10.1007/s12187-014-9248-4.

Ansell, Nicola. 2014. "Challenging Empowerment: AIDS-Affected Southern African Children and the Need for a Multi-Level Relational Approach." *Journal of Health Psychology* 19 (1): 22–33.

Anthony, S. 1972. *The Discovery of Death in Childhood and After*, 2nd ed. New York: Basic Books.

Ariès, Philippe. 1981. *The Hour of Our Death*. New York: Alfred Knopf.

Armstrong, David. 1995. "The Rise of Surveillance Medicine." *Sociology of Health & Illness* 17 (3): 393–404.

Atwool, Nicola. 1999. "New Zealand Children in the 1990s: Beneficiaries of New Right Economic Policy?" *Children & Society* 13 (5): 380–393.

Baker, Michael G., Lucy Telfar Barnard, Amanda Kvalsvig, Ayesha Verrall, Jane Zhang, Michael Keall, Nick Wilson, Teresa Wall, and Philippa Howden-Chapman. 2012. "Increasing Incidence of Serious Infectious Diseases and Inequalities in New Zealand: A National Epidemiological Study." *Lancet* 379 (9821): 1112–1119.

Baker, Michael G., Anne McNicholas, Nicholas Garrett, Nicholas Jones, Joanna Stewart, Vivien Koberstein, and Diana R. Lennon. 2000. "Household Crowding a Major Risk Factor for Epidemic Meningococcal Disease in Auckland Children." *Pediatric Infectious Disease Journal* 19 (10): 983–990.

Barber, Brian K. 2013. "Annual Research Review: The Experience of Youth with Political Conflict—Challenging Notions of Resilience and Encouraging Research Refinement." *Journal of Child Psychology and Psychiatry* 54 (4): 461–473.

Barbera, Mattia. 2011. "Three Pacific Countries and Auckland . . . the Capital of the Pacific?" Social and Economic Research Team Research, Investigations & Monitoring Unit, Auckland Council. Available from http://knowledgeauckland.org.nz/assets/publications/Three_Pacific_Countries_and_Auckland__the_Capital_of_the_Pacific_.pdf.

Barraclough, Breanna. 2017. "Five Years On: Lunchbox Differences in Decile 1 and Decile 10 Schools." *Newshub*, December 9, 2017, sec. NZ, http://www.newshub.co.nz/home/new-zealand/2017/09/five-years-on-lunchbox-differences-in-decile-1-and-decile-10-schools.html.

Becker, Ernest. 1973. *The Denial of Death*. New York: Free Press.

Belich, James. 2001. *Paradise Reforged: A History of the New Zealanders from the 1880s to the Year 2000*. Honolulu: University of Hawai'i Press.

Bell, A. C., and W. R. Parnell. 1996. "Nutritient Intakes of Tongan and Tokelauan Children Living in New Zealand." *New Zealand Medical Journal* 109 (1034): 435–38.

Bell, Avril. 2004. "Relating Māori and Pākehā: The Politics of Indigenous and Settler Identities." Ph.D. Dissertation, Massey University.

Birch, Leann Lipps, Linda McPhee, B. C. Shoba, Lois Steinberg, and Ruth Krehbiel. 1987. "'Clean Up Your Plate': Effects of Child Feeding Practices on the Conditioning of Meal Size." *Learning and Motivation* 18 (3): 301–317.

Blank, Anton, Carla Houkamau, and Hautahi Kingi. 2016. "Unconscious Bias and Education: A Comparative Study of Māori and African American Students." Oranui Diversity Leadership. Available from https://apo.org.au/node/65536.

Bluebond-Langner, Myra. 1978. *The Private Worlds of Dying Children*. Princeton, NJ: Princeton University Press.

———. 2000. *In the Shadow of Illness: Parents and Siblings of the Chronically Ill Child*. Princeton, NJ: Princeton University Press.

Boas, Franz. 1974. "The Instability of Human Types." In *The Shaping of American Anthropology 1883–1911: A Franz Boas Reader*, ed. George W. Stocking, 214–218. New York: Basic Books.

Bogin, Barry A., and James Loucky. 1997. "Plasticity, Political Economy, and Physical Growth Status of Guatemala Maya Children Living in the United States." *American Journal of Physical Anthropology* 102: 17–32.

Bolin, Inge. 2006. *Growing Up in a Culture of Respect: Child Rearing in Highland Peru*. Austin: University of Texas Press.

Bonanno, George A., and Erica D. Diminich. 2013. "Annual Research Review: Positive Adjustment to Adversity: Trajectories of Minimal-Impact Resilience and Emergent Resilience." *Journal of Child Psychology and Psychiatry* 54 (4): 378–401.

Borneman, John. 2009. "Fieldwork Experience, Collaboration, and Interlocution: The 'Meta-physics of Presence' in Encounters with the Syrian Mukhabarat." In *Being There: The Fieldwork Encounter and the Making of Truth*, ed. John Borneman and Abdellah Hammoudi, 237–258. Berkeley: University of California Press.

Borneman, John, and Abdellah Hammoudi, eds. 2009. *Being There: The Fieldwork Encounter and the Making of Truth*. Berkeley: University of California Press.

Borrell, Belinda. 2005. "Living in the City Ain't So Bad: Cultural Identity for Young Maori in South Auckland." In *New Zealand Identities: Departures and Destinations*, ed. James H. Liu, Tim McCreanor, Tracey McIntosh, and Teresia Teaiwa, 369–400. Wellington: Victoria University Press.

Boston, Jonathan, and Simon Chapple. 2014. *Child Poverty in New Zealand*. Wellington: Bridget Williams Books Limited.

Bourdieu, Pierre. 1977. *Outline of a Theory of Practice*. Cambridge: Cambridge University Press.

——. 1984. *Distinction: A Social Critique of the Judgement of Taste*. Cambridge, MA: Harvard University Press.

——. 1986. "The Forms of Capital." In *Handbook of Theory and Research for the Sociology of Education*, ed. J. Richardson. New York: Macmillan.

Bourgois, Philippe. 1995. "In Search of Respect: Selling Crack in el Barrio." *Structural Analysis in the Social Sciences*. Cambridge: Cambridge University Press.

Boyd, Sally. 2011. "Educating Healthy Citizens in New Zealand Schools: Students Leading the Way." Annual Meeting of the American Educational Research Association, New Orleans. Available from http://www.nzcer.org.nz/system/files/educating-healthy-citizens.pdf.

Boyden, Jo, C. Eyber, T. Feeny, and C. Scott. 2004. *Children and Poverty. Part II. Voices of Children: Experiences and Perceptions from Belarus, Bolivia, India, Kenya and Sierra Leone*. Children in Poverty Series. Richmond, VA: Christian Children's Fund.

Boyden, Jo, and Gillian Mann. 2005. "Children's Risk, Resilience, and Coping in Extreme Situations." In *Handbook for Working with Children and Youth: Pathways to Resilience across Cultures and Contexts*, ed. Michael Ungar, 3–26. Thousand Oaks, CA: Sage.

Brady, Ivan, ed. 1976. *Transaction in Kinship: Adoption and Fosterage in Oceania*. ASAO Monograph No. 4. Honolulu: University of Hawai'i Press.

Briggs, Jean L. 1970. *Never in Anger: Portrait of an Eskimo Family*. Cambridge, MA: Harvard University Press.

——. 1979. "Aspects of Inuit Value Socialization." Canadian Ethnology Service paper no. 56. Ottawa: National Museums of Canada.

——. 1998. *Inuit Morality Play: The Emotional Education of a Three-Year-Old*. New Haven, CT: Yale University Press.

Brison, Karen J. 2014. *Children, Social Class, and Education: Shifting Identities in Fiji*. Culture, Mind, and Society. London: Palgrave Macmillan.

Broch, Harald Beyer. 1990. *Growing Up Agreeably: Bonerate Childhood Observed*. University of Hawai'i Press.

Bronfenbrenner, U. 1979. *The Ecology of Human Development: Experiments by Nature and Design*. Cambridge, MA: Harvard University Press.

Broszormenyi-Nagy, I., and G. M. Spark. 1973. *Invisible Loyalties: Reciprocity in Intergenerational Family Therapy*. Hagerstown, MD: Harper & Row.

Bryant, Penelope A., Roy Robins-Browne, Jonathan R. Carapetis, and Nigel Curtis. 2009. "Some of the People, Some of the Time: Susceptibility to Acute Rheumatic Fever." *Circulation* 119 (5): 742–753.

Buckingham, David. 2011. *The Material Child: Growing Up in Consumer Culture*. Cambridge: Polity Press.

Burrow, Alicia. 2015. "Kids' Lunch Should Come from Parents—Government." *Stuff*, March 24, 2015. Available from http://www.stuff.co.nz/national/politics/67483679/kids-lunch-should-come-from-parents—government.

Burrows, Lisette, and Jan Wright. 2007. "Prescribing Practices: Shaping Healthy Children in Schools." *International Journal of Children's Rights* 15: 83–98.

Bynum, L., T. Griffin, D. L. Riding, K. S. Wynkoop, R. F. Anda, V. J. Edwards, T. W. Strine, Y. Liu, L. R. McKnight-Eily, and J. B. Croft. 2010. "Adverse Childhood Experiences Reported by Adults— Five States, 2009." *Morbidity and Mortality Weekly Report* 59 (49): 1609–1613.

Campbell, Catherine, Louise Andersen, Alice Mutsikiwa, Claudius Madanhire, Morten Skovdal, Constance Nyamukapa, and Simon Gregson. 2015. "Re-thinking Children's Agency in Extreme Hardship: Zimbabwean Children's Draw-and-Write about Their HIV-Affected Peers." *Health & Place* 31: 54–64.

Carapetis, Jonathan R., B. J. Currie, and J. D. Mathews. 2000. "Cumulative Incidence of Rheumatic Fever in an Endemic Region: A Guide to the Susceptibility of the Population?" *Epidemiology and Infection* 124 (2): 239–244.

Carapetis, Jonathan R., Andrew C. Steer, E. Kim Mulholland, and Martin Weber. 2005. "The Global Burden of Group A Streptococcal Diseases." *Lancet Infectious Diseases* 5 (11): 685–94, https://doi.org/10.1016/S1473-3099(05)70267-X.

Carroll, Vern, ed. 1970. *Adoption in Eastern Oceania*. ASAO Monograph No. 1. Honolulu: University of Hawai'i Press.

Caspi, Avshalom, Renate M. Houts, Daniel W. Belsky, Honalee Harrington, Sean Hogan, Sandhya Ramrakha, Richie Poulton, and Terrie E. Moffitt. 2016. "Childhood Forecasting of a Small Segment of the Population with Large Economic Burden." *Nature Human Behaviour* 1 (1): s41562-016-0005-016, https://doi.org/10.1038/s41562-016-0005.

Chapin, Bambi. 2014. *Childhood in a Sri Lankin Village: Shaping Hierarchy and Desire*. New Brunswick, N.J.: Rutgers University Press.

Cheer, Tarin, Robin Kearns, and Laurence Murphy. 2002. "Housing Policy, Poverty, and Culture: 'Discounting' Decisions among Pacific Peoples in Auckland, New Zealand." *Environment and Planning C: Government and Policy* 20 (4): 497–516, https://doi.org/10.1068/c04r.

Cheney, Kristen E. 2017. *Crying for Our Elders: African Orphanhood in the Age of HIV and AIDS*. Chicago: University of Chicago Press.

Christensen, Pia. 1999. "Towards an Anthropology of Childhood Sickness: An Ethnographic Study of Danish Schoolchildren." Doctoral thesis, University of Hull.

———. 2000. "Childhood and the Cultural Constitution of Vulnerable Bodies." In *Body, Childhood and Society*, ed. A. Prout. London: Palgrave Macmillan.

———. 2004. "Children's Participation in Ethnographic Research: Issues of Power and Representation." *Children & Society* 18: 165–176.

Christensen, Pia, Allison James, and Chris Jenks. 2001. "'All We Needed to Do Was Blow the Whistle': Children's Embodiment of Time." *Explorations in Sociology* 61: 201–222.

Christensen, Pia, and Alan Prout. 2002. "Working with Ethical Symmetry in Social Research with Children." *Childhood* 9 (4): 477–497.

Clark, Cindy Dell. 1998. *Flights of Fancy, Leaps of Faith: Children's Myths in Contemporary America*. Chicago: University of Chicago Press.

———. 2003. *In Sickness and in Play: Children Coping with Chronic Illness*. New Brunswick, NJ: Rutgers University Press.

Cleland, Alison. 2013. "Children's and Young People's Participation in Legal Proceedings in Aotearoa New Zealand: Significant Challenges Lie Ahead." *New Zealand Law Review* 2013 (3), 483–504.

———. 2016. "A Long Lesson in Humility? The Inability of Child Care Law to Promote the Well-Being of Children." In *Implementing Article 3 of the United Nations Convention on the Rights of the Child*, ed. Elaine E. Sutherland and L-A Barnes, 131–146. Cambridge: Cambridge University Press.

Clifford, James, and George E. Marcus. 1986. *Writing Culture: The Poetics and Politics of Ethnography: A School of American Research Advanced Seminar*. Berkeley: University of California Press.

Colls, Rachel, and Kathrin Hörschelmann. 2009. "Introduction: Contested Bodies of Childhood and Youth." In *Contested Bodies of Childhood and Youth*, ed. K. Hörschelmann and R. Colls, 1–21. London: Palgrave Macmillan.

Colman, Ian, Mila Kingsbury, Murray Weeks, Anushka Ataullahjan, Marc-André Bélair, Jennifer Dykxhoorn, Katie Hynes, Alexandra Loro, Michael S. Martin, Kiyuri Naicker, et al. 2014. "Cartoons Kill: Casualties in Animated Recreational Theater in an Objective Observational New Study of Kids' Introduction to Loss of Life." *BMJ* 349: g7184.

Connolly, Paul. 2004. *Boys and Schooling in the Early Years*. London: Routledge Falmer.

Cooper, Christopher S., Chadi T. Abousally, J. C. Austin, Margaret A. Boyt, and Charles E. Hawtrey. 2003. "Do Public Schools Teach Voiding Dysfunction? Results of an Elementary School Teacher Survey." *The Journal of Urology* 170 (3): 956–958.

Corsaro, William A. 1979. "'We're Friends, Right?': Children's Use of Access Rituals in a Nursery School." *Language in Society*, 315–336.

———. 1992. "Interpretive Reproduction in Children's Peer Cultures." *Social Psychology Quarterly* 55 (2): 160–177, https://doi.org/10.2307/2786944.

———. 2015. *The Sociology of Childhood*, 4th ed. Thousand Oaks, CA: Sage Publications.

Counts, Dorothy Ayers, and David R. Counts, eds. 1985. *Aging and Its Transformations: Moving toward Death in Pacific Societies*. Pittsburgh, PA: University of Pittsburgh Press.

Craig, Elsdon. 1982. *Breakwater Against the Tide: A History of Papakura City and Districts*. Auckland: Ray Richards.

Crimes (Substituted Section 59) Amendment Act 2007, http://www.legislation.govt.nz/act/public/2007/0018/latest/DLM407664.html.

Crossley, Nick. 2001. "The Phenomenological Habitus and Its Construction." *Theory and Society* 30 (1): 81–120.

Csordas, Thomas J. 1993. "Somatic Modes of Attention." *Cultural Anthropology* 8 (2): 135–156.

Cuddy-Casey, Maria, and Helen Orvaschel. 1997. "Children's Understanding of Death in Relation to Child Suicidality and Homicidality." *Clinical Psychology Review* 17 (1): 33–45, https://doi.org/10.1016/S0272-7358(96)00044-X.

Cushman, Penni. 2008. "Health Promoting Schools: A New Zealand Perspective." *Pastoral Care in Education* 26 (4): 231–241, https://doi.org/10.1080/02643940802472163.

Dansey, Harry. 1975. "A View of Death." In *Te Ao Hurihuri—the World Moves on: Aspects of Maoritanga*, ed. Michael King, 173–189. Wellington: Hicks Smith.

Das, Veena. 1989. "Voices of Children." *Daedalus* 118 (4): 262.

———. 2015. *In Pursuit of the Good Life: Aspiration and Suicide in Globalizing South India*. Hoboken, NJ: Wiley-Blackwell.

Davies, Hayley. 2015. *Understanding Children's Personal Lives and Relationships*. Palgrave Macmillan Studies in Family and Intimate Life. London: Palgrave Macmillan.

———. 2017. "Embodied and Sensory Encounters: Death, Bereavement and Remembering in Children's Family and Personal Lives." *Children's Geographies*, 1–13.

Davies, Matthew. 2008. "A Childish Culture? Shared Understandings, Agency and Intervention: An Anthropological Study of Street Children in Northwest Kenya." *Childhood* 15 (3): 309–330, https://doi.org/10.1177/0907568208091666.

Davis, Susan Schaefer, and Douglas A. Davis. 1989. *Adolescence in a Moroccan Town: Making Social Sense*. New Brunswick, NJ: Rutgers University Press.

De Certeau, M. 1988. *The Practice of Everyday Life*, vol. 1. Berkeley: University of California Press.

Dei, George Jerry Sefa. 1997. *Reconstructing "Dropout": A Critical Ethnography of the Dynamics of Black Students' Disengagement from School*. Toronto: University of Toronto Press.

Desjarlais, Robert. 1992. *Body and Emotion: The Aesthetics of Illness and Healing in the Nepal Himalayas*. Philadelphia: University of Pennsylvania Press.

Desjarlais, Robert, and Jason C. Throop. 2011. "Phenomenological Approaches in Anthropology." *Annual Review of Anthropology* 40: 87–102.

Dominguez, Virginia. 2016. "Introduction: Ethics, Work and Life—Individual Struggles and Professional 'Comfort Zones' in Anthropology." In *Anthropological Ethics in Context: An Ongoing Dialogue*, ed. Dena Plemmons and Alex W. Barker, 9–21. Walnut Creek, CA: Left Coast Press.

D'Souza, Amanda J. 2017. "The Rise of Child-Friendly Public Policy in Aotearoa." Conference paper, Fourth Childhood Studies Colloquium, November 13, 2017, Victoria University, Wellington.

Duncanson, M., G. Oben, M. A. McGee, S. Morris, A. Wicken, and J. Simpson. 2017. "Child Poverty Monitor: Technical Report 2017." New Zealand Child and Youth Epidemiology Service. Available from http://hdl.handle.net/10523/7775.

Dunsford, Deborah, Julie Park, Judith Littleton, Ward Friesen, Phyllis Herda, Pat Neuwelt, and Jennifer Hand. 2011. *Better Lives: The Struggle for Health of Transnational Pacific Peoples in New Zealand, 1950–2000*. Research in Anthropology & Linguistics, No. 9. Auckland: Department of Anthropology, University of Auckland.

Durham, Deborah. 2008. "Apathy and Agency: The Romance of Agency and Youth in Botswana." In *Figuring the Future: Globalization and the Temporalities of Children and Youth*, ed. Jennifer Cole and Deborah Durham, 151–178. Santa Fe: School for Advanced Research Press.

Durie, Mason H. 2001. *Mauri Ora: The Dynamics of Māori Health*. Auckland: Oxford University Press.

Durie-Hall, Donna, and Joan Metge. 1992. "Kua Tutū Te Puehu, Kia Mau: Maori Aspirations and Family Law." In *Family Law Policy in New Zealand*, ed. Mark Henaghan and Bill Atkin. Auckland: Oxford University Press.

Easton, Brian. 1980. *Social Policy and the Welfare State in New Zealand*. Auckland: George Allen & Unwin.

Eggerman, Mark, and Catherine Panter-Brick. 2010. "Suffering, Hope, and Entrapment: Resilience and Cultural Values in Afghanistan." *Social Science & Medicine* 71: 71–83, https://doi.org/10.1016/j.socscimed.2010.03.023.

Elias, Norbert. 1978. *The Civilizing Process*. Oxford: Blackwell.

———. 1982. *The Civilizing Process*, vol. 2. Oxford: Blackwell.

Elizabeth, Vivienne, and Wendy Larner. 2009. "Racializing the 'Social Development' State: Investing in Children in Aotearoa/New Zealand." *Social Politics: International Studies in Gender, State & Society* 16 (1): 132–158, https://doi.org/10.1093/sp/jxp001.

Ellison-Loschmann, L, P. K. Pattemore, M. I. Asher, T. O. Clayton, J. Crane, P. Ellwood, R. J. Mackay, E. A. Mitchell, C. Moyes, and N. Pearce. 2009. "Ethnic Differences in Time

Trends in Asthma Prevalence in New Zealand: ISAAC Phases I and III." *International Journal of Tuberculosis and Lung Disease* 13: 775–782.

Farmer, Paul. 2003. *Pathologies of Power: Health, Human Rights, and the New War on the Poor*, vol. 4. Berkeley: University of California Press.

———. 2004. "An Anthropology of Structural Violence." *Current Anthropology* 45 (3): 305–325, https://doi.org/10.1086/382250.

Felitti, Vincent J., Robert F. Anda, Dale Nordenberg, David F. Williamson, Alison M. Spitz, Valerie Edwards, Mary P. Koss, and James S. Marks. 1998. "Relationship of Childhood Abuse and Household Dysfunction to Many of the Leading Causes of Death in Adults." *American Journal of Preventive Medicine* 14 (4): 245–58, https://doi.org/10.1016/S0749-3797(98)00017-8.

Fergusson, David M., Joseph M. Boden, and L. John Horwood. 2015. "From Evidence to Policy: Findings from the Christchurch Health and Development Study." *Australian & New Zealand Journal of Criminology* 48 (3): 386–408, https://doi.org/10.1177/0004865815589827.

Fergusson, David M., L. John Horwood, and Joseph M. Boden. 2008. "The Transmission of Social Inequality: Examination of the Linkages between Family Socioeconomic Status in Childhood and Educational Achievement in Young Adulthood." *Research in Social Stratification and Mobility* 26 (3): 277–295, https://doi.org/10.1016/j.rssm.2008.05.001.

Fergusson, David M., and Lianne J. Woodward. 2000. "Family Socioeconomic Status at Birth and Rates of University Participation." *New Zealand Journal of Educational Studies* 35 (1): 25–36.

Fine, Gary Alan, and Kent L. Sandstrom. 1988. *Knowing Children: Participant Observation with Minors*. Newbury Park, CA: Sage.

Fitzmaurice, Luke. 2017. "Children's Voices in System Reform: A Case Study on Children and Young People's Participation within the Modernisation of Child, Youth and Family." *Aotearoa New Zealand Social Work* 29 (1): 41.

Fleming, Theresa M., Terryann Clark, Simon Denny, Pat Bullen, Sue Crengle, Roshini Peiris-John, Elizabeth Robinson, Fiona V. Rossen, Janie Sheridan, and Mathijs Lucassen. 2014. "Stability and Change in the Mental Health of New Zealand Secondary School Students 2007–2012: Results from the National Adolescent Health Surveys." *Australian and New Zealand Journal of Psychiatry* 48 (5): 472–480, https://doi.org/10.1177/0004867413514489.

Flinn, Mark V. 1999. "Family Environment, Stress, and Health during Childhood." In *Hormones, Health, and Behavior: A Socio-Ecological and Lifespan Perspective*, ed. Catherine Panter-Brick, 105–138. Cambridge: Cambridge University Press.

———. 2011. "Social Inequalities, Family Relationships, and Child Health." In *Biosocial Foundations of Family Processes*, ed. Alan Booth, Susan M. McHale, and Nancy S. Landale, 205–220. New York: Springer.

Flinn, Mark V., and Barry G. England. 1995. "Childhood Stress and Family Environment." *Current Anthropology* 36: 854–866.

———. 1997. "Social Economics of Childhood Glucocorticoid Stress Response and Health." *American Journal of Physical Anthropology* 102: 33–53.

Flinn, Mark V., C. V. Ward, and R. Noone. 2005. "Hormones and the Human Family." In *Handbook of Evolutionary Psychology*, ed. D. Buss, 552–580. New York: Wiley.

Fomon, Samuel J., L. J. Filer, N. A. Thomas, Thomas A. Anderson, and Steven E. Nelson. 1975. "Influence of Formula Concentration on Caloric Intake and Growth of Normal Infants." *Acta Paediatrica* 64 (2): 172–181.

"Fonterra Milk for Schools." n.d. Web page accessed February 20, 2018. Available from www.fonterramilkforschools.com.

Forbes, Mihingarangi (presenter). 2017. "The Hui: Ngā Mōrehu—Survivors of State Abuse."
    The Hui, episode 3. Television documentary, aired April 9, 2017.
Foucault, Michel. 1979. *Discipline and Punish: The Birth of the Prison.* New York: Vintage Books.
———. 1980. *Power/Knowledge: Selected Interviews and Other Writings, 1972–1977.* Brighton,
    Sussex, U.K.: Harvester Press.
———. 1990. *The History of Sexuality.* London: Penguin Books.
France, Alan. 2012. "'It's All in the Brain': Science and the 'New' Construction of the Youth
    Problem in New Zealand." *New Zealand Sociology* 27 (2): 76–95.
Frankenberg, Ronald. 1980. "Medical Anthropology and Development: A Theoretical
    Perspective." *Social Science & Medicine* 14B: 197–207.
———. 1990. "Disease, Literature and the Body in the Era of AIDS: A Preliminary Explora-
    tion." *Sociology of Health & Illness* 12 (3): 351–360.
Frankenberg, Ronald, Ian Robinson, and Amber Delahooke. 2000. "Countering Essentialism
    in Behavioural Social Science: The Example of 'the Vulnerable Child' Ethnographically
    Examined." *Sociological Review* 48 (4): 586–611.
Freund, Peter. 1982. *The Civilized Body: Social Domination, Control, and Health.* Philadelphia:
    Temple University Press.
Frisancho, A. Roberto. 1993. *Human Adaptation and Accommodation.* Ann Arbor: University
    of Michigan Press.
Gagné, Natacha. 2013. *Being Māori in the City: Indigenous Everyday Life in Auckland.* Toronto:
    University of Toronto Press.
Gallacher, Lesley-Anne, and Michael Gallagher. 2008. "Methodological Immaturity in Child-
    hood Research? Thinking through Participatory Methods." *Childhood* 15 (4): 499–516.
Galtung, Johan. 1969. "Violence, Peace, and Peace Research." *Journal of Peace Research* 6 (3):
    167–191.
Garnier, Pascale. 2015. "Between Young Children and Adults: Practical Logic in Families'
    Lives." In *Childhood with Bourdieu,* ed. Leena Alanen, E. Brooker, and Berry Mayall,
    57–77. London: Palgrave Macmillan.
Geertz, Clifford. 1973. *The Interpretation of Cultures: Selected Essays.* New York: Basic Books.
Geurts, Kathryn. 2003. *Culture and the Senses: Bodily Ways of Knowing in an African Commu-
    nity.* Berkeley: University of California Press.
Gibb, Sheree J., David M. Fergusson, and L. John Horwood. 2012. "Childhood Family Income
    and Life Outcomes in Adulthood: Findings from a 30-Year Longitudinal Study in New
    Zealand." *Social Science & Medicine* 74 (12): 1979–1986, https://doi.org/10.1016/j.socscimed
    .2012.02.028.
Giddens, Nagy. 1979. *Central Problems in Social Theory: Action, Structure and Contradiction in
    Social Analysis.* Berkeley: University of California Press.
Gilbert, Jane. 2005. *Educational Issues for Communities Affected by Transience and Residential
    Mobility: Report on Phase 1 (2003–2004).* Wellington: New Zealand Council for Educa-
    tional Research.
Gilbert, Leah K., Matthew J. Breiding, Melissa T. Merrick, William W. Thompson, Derek C.
    Ford, Satvinder S. Dhingra, and Sharyn E. Parks. 2015. "Childhood Adversity and Adult
    Chronic Disease: An Update from Ten States and the District of Columbia, 2010." *Amer-
    ican Journal of Preventive Medicine* 48 (3): 345–349, https://doi.org/10.1016/j.amepre
    .2014.09.006.
Ginsburg, Herbert, and Sylvia Opper. 1988. *Piaget's Theory of Intellectual Development.* Engle-
    wood Cliffs, NJ: Prentice-Hall.
Gold, Raymond L. 1958. "Roles in Sociological Field Observations." *Social Forces* 36 (3):
    217–223.

Goode, David A. 1986. "Kids, Culture and Innocents." *Human Studies* 9 (1): 83–106.

Grace, Patricia. 1986. *Potiki*. Auckland: Penguin Books.

Grant, C. C. 1999. "Pneumonia in Children: Becoming Harder to Ignore." *New Zealand Medical Journal* 112 (1095): 345–347.

Green, James W. 2012. *Beyond the Good Death: The Anthropology of Modern Dying*. Philadelphia: University of Pennsylvania Press.

Gross, R., B. Landfried, and S. Herman. 1996. "Height and Weight as a Reflection of the Nutritional Situation of School-Aged Children Working and Living in the Streets of Jakarta." *Social Science & Medicine* 43: 453–458.

Haggerty, R. J. 1986. "Stress and Illness in Children." *Bulletin of the New York Academy of Medicine* 62 (7): 707–18.

Hardy, I. R. B., Diana R. Lennon, and E. A. Mitchell. 1987. "Measles Epidemic in Auckland 1984–85." *New Zealand Medical Journal* 100: 273–275.

Harris, Ricci, Donna M. Cormack, and James Stanley. 2013. "The Relationship between Socially-Assigned Ethnicity, Health and Experience of Racial Discrimination for Māori: Analysis of the 2006/07 New Zealand Health Survey." *BMC Public Health* 13 (1): 844.

Harris, Ricci, Martin Tobias, Mona Jeffreys, Kiri Waldegrave, Saffron Karlsen, and James Nazroo. 2006. "Racism and Health: The Relationship between Experience of Racial Discrimination and Health in New Zealand." *Social Science & Medicine* 63 (6): 1428–1441.

Hastrup, Kirsten. 1993. "Hunger and the Hardness of Facts." *Man*, 727–739.

Havea, Jione. 2013. "Death Roots: Musings of a Pacific Island Native." In *Pacific Identities and Well-Being: Cross-Cultural Perspectives*, edited by Margaret Agee, Tracey McIntosh, Philip Culbertson, and Cabrini 'Ofa Makasiale, 175–85. New York: Rutledge.

Heath, Shirley Brice. 1983. *Ways with Words: Language, Life and Work in Communities and Classrooms*. Cambridge: Cambridge University Press.

Hecht, Tobias. 1998. *At Home in the Street: Street Children of Northeast Brazil*. Cambridge: Cambridge University Press.

Henare, Manuka, Adrienne Puckey, and Amber Nicholson. 2011. "He Ara Hou: The Pathway Forward Getting It Right for Aotearoa New Zealand's Māori and Pasifika Children." Auckland: Mira Szászy Research Centre, University of Auckland.

Herman, C. P., and J. Polivy. 2008. "External Cues in the Control of Food Intake in Humans: The Sensory-Normative Distinction." *Physiology & Behavior* 94 (5): 722–728.

Heyman, Melvin B. 2006. "Lactose Intolerance in Infants, Children, and Adolescents." *Pediatrics* 118 (3): 1279–1286, https://doi.org/10.1542/peds.2006-1721.

Holmes, Lowell. 1974. *Samoan Village*. New York: Holt, Rinehart & Winston.

Hörschelmann, Kathrin, and Rachel Colls, eds. 2009. *Contested Bodies of Childhood and Youth*. London: Palgrave Macmillan.

Horton, Sarah, and Judith C. Barker. 2010. "Stigmatized Biologies." *Medical Anthropology Quarterly* 24 (2): 199–219.

Howden-Chapman, Philippa, Gina Pene, Julian Crane, Robyn Green, Loi Iupati, Ian Prior, and Ioane Teao. 2000. "Open Houses and Closed Rooms: Tokelau Housing in New Zealand." *Health Education and Behavior* 27: 351–362.

Howes, David. 2006. "Charting the Sensorial Revolution." *The Senses and Society* 1 (1): 113–128.

Hunleth, Jean. 2011. "Beyond on or with: Questioning Power Dynamics and Knowledge Production in 'Child-Oriented' Research Methodology." *Childhood* 18 (1): 81–93.

———. 2017. *Children as Caregivers: The Global Fight Against Tuberculosis and HIV in Zambia*. New Brunswick, NJ: Rutgers University Press.

Husserl, Edmund. 1962. *Ideas: General Introduction to Pure Phenomenology.* New York: Collier.

Jacob, Juanita Emily. 2011. "Maori Children: Conceptions of Death and Tangihanga". Master's thesis, University of Waikato.

Jaine, Richard, Michael G. Baker, and Kamalesh Venugopal. 2008. "Epidemiology of Acute Rheumatic Fever in New Zealand 1996–2005." *Journal of Paediatrics and Child Health* 44 (10): 564–571, https://doi.org/10.1111/j.1440-1754.2008.01384.x.

———. 2011. "Acute Rheumatic Fever Associated with Household Crowding in a Developed Country," *Pediatric Infectious Disease Journal* 30 (4): 315–319.

James, Allison. 1993. *Childhood Identities: Self and Social Relationships in the Experience of the Child.* Edinburgh: Edinburgh University Press.

———. 2000. "Embodied Being (s): Understanding the Self and the Body in Childhood." In *The Body, Childhood and Society,* ed. Alan Prout, 19–37. London: Palgrave Macmillan.

———. 2001. "Ethnography in the Study of Children and Childhood." In *Handbook of Ethnography,* ed. Paul Atkinson, Amanda Coffey, Sara Delamont, John Lofland, and Lyn Lofland, 246–257. Thousand Oaks, CA: Sage.

———. 2013. *Socialising Children.* London: Palgrave Macmillan.

James, Allison, Chris Jenks, and Alan Prout. 1998. *Theorizing Childhood.* Cambridge: Polity Press.

James, Allison, and Alan Prout. 1990. *Constructing and Reconstructing Childhood: Contemporary Issues in the Sociological Study of Childhood.* New York: Falmer Press.

Jasanoff, Sheila. 2004. *States of Knowledge: The Coproduction of Science and the Social Order.* London: Routledge.

Jenkins, Richard. 1982. "Pierre Bourdieu and the Reproduction of Determinism." *Sociology* 16 (2): 270–281.

Johnston, Kirsty. 2015. "Education Investigation: The Great Divide." *New Zealand Herald,* November 4, 2015, http://www.nzherald.co.nz/nz/news/article.cfm?c_id=1&objectid=11539592.

Johnston, Kirsty, and Chris Knox. 2017. "Childhood Diseases in the Land of Milk and Poverty." New Zealand Herald, August 8, 2017, http://www.nzherald.co.nz/nz/news/article.cfm?c_id=1&objectid=11913334.

Kaeppler, Adrienne L. 1978. "Me'a Faka' Eiki: Tongan Funerals in a Changing Society." In *The Changing Pacific,* edited by H.E. Maude, 174–202. Melbourne: Oxford University Press.

Kastenbaum, Robert, and Lynn Fox. 2008. "Do Imaginary Companions Die? An Exploratory Study." *OMEGA* 56 (2): 123–152.

Katriel, Tamar. 1987. "'Bexibùdim!'": Ritualized Sharing among Israeli Children." *Language in Society* 16 (03): 305–320.

———. 1988. "Haxlàfot: Rules and Strategies in Children's Swapping Exchanges." *Research on Language & Social Interaction* 22 (1–4): 157–178.

Kearns, Robin A., and Damian C. A. Collins. 2000. "New Zealand Children's Health Camps: Therapeutic Landscapes Meet the Contract State." *Social Science & Medicine* 51 (7): 1047–1059.

Keddell, Emily. 2018. "The Vulnerable Child in Neoliberal Contexts: The Construction of Children in the Aotearoa New Zealand Child Protection Reforms." *Childhood* 25 (1): 93–108, https://doi.org/10.1177/0907568217727591.

Kenner, Charmian, Mahera Ruby, John Jessel, Eve Gregory, and Tahera Arju. 2007. "Intergenerational Learning between Children and Grandparents in East London." *Journal of Early Childhood Research* 5 (3): 219–243, https://doi.org/10.1177/1476718X07080471.

King, Michael. 1985. *Being Pakeha: An Encounter with New Zealand and the Maori Renaissance.* Auckland: Hodder and Stoughton.

Kloos, Peter. 1969. "Role Conflicts in Social Fieldwork." *Current Anthropology* 10 (5): 509–512.

Korbin, Jill E., and Pamela Zahorik. 1985. "Childhood, Health, and Illness: Beliefs and Behaviors of Urban American Schoolchildren." *Medical Anthropology* 9 (4): 337–353.

Kraftl, Peter. 2013. "Beyond 'Voice,' beyond 'Agency,' beyond 'Politics'? Hybrid Childhoods and Some Critical Reflections on Children's Emotional Geographies." *Emotion, Space and Society* 9: 13–23.

Kramer, Karen. 2005. *Maya Children: Helpers at the Farm.* Cambridge, MA: Harvard University Press.

Krieger, Nancy. 2005. "Embodiment: A Conceptual Glossary for Epidemiology." *Journal of Epidemiology and Community Health* 59: 350.

Lancy, David F. 2012. "Unmasking Children's Agency." SSWA Faculty Publications, paper 277, http://digitalcommons.usu.edu/sswa_facpubs/277/.

Lansdown, Gerison. 2010. "The Realisation of Children's Participation Rights." In *A Handbook of Children and Young People's Participation: Perspectives from Theory and Practice*, ed. B. Percy-Smith and N. Thomas, 11–23. London: Routledge.

Larner, Wendy. 1997. "'A Means to an End': Neoliberalism and State Processes in New Zealand." *Studies in Political Economy* 52 (1): 7–38.

———. 2000. "Post-Welfare State Governance: Towards a Code of Social and Family Responsibility." *Social Politics: International Studies in Gender, State & Society* 7 (2): 244–265, https://doi.org/10.1093/sp/7.2.244.

Layne, Christopher M., Jared S. Warren, Patricia J. Watson, and Arieh Y. Shalev. 2007. "Risk, Vulnerability, Resistance, and Resilience: Towards an Integrative Conceptualization of Posttraumatic Adaptation." In *Handbook of PTSD: Science and Practice*, edited by Matthew Friedman, Terence Keane, and Patricia Resnick, 497–520. New York: Guilford Press.

Lee, Nick. 2013. *Childhood and Biopolitics: Climate Change, Life Processes and Human Futures.* London: Palgrave Macmillan.

Lee, Nick, and Johanna Motzkau. 2011. "Navigating the Bio-Politics of Childhood." *Childhood* 18 (1): 7–19.

Lennon, Diana R., B. Gellin, D. Hood, D. T. Leach, G. M. Woods, P. Williams, S. Thakur, and D. Crombie. 1993. "Control of Epidemic Group A Meningococcal Disease in Auckland." *New Zealand Medical Journal* 106 (948): 3–6.

Lennon, Diana R., D. Martin, E. Wong, and L. R. Taylor. 1988. "Longitudinal Study of Post-streptococcal Disease in Auckland: Rheumatic Fever, Glomerulonephritis, Epidemiology and M Typing 1981–86." *New Zealand Medical Journal* 101 (847 Pt. 2): 396–398.

Lennon, Diana R., Briar Peat, Melissa Kerdemelidis, Norman Sharpe, and Rachel Liddel. 2014. "New Zealand Guidelines for Rheumatic Fever Group A Streptococcal Sore Throat Management Guideline: 2014 Update." Heart Foundation New Zealand, Auckland. Available from http://www.ttophs.govt.nz/vdb/document/1056.

LeVine, Robert A. 1977. "Child Rearing as Cultural Adaptation." In *Culture and Infancy*, ed. P. Herbert Leiderman, Steven R. Tulkin, and Anne H. Rosenfeld, 15–27. New York: Academic Press.

———. 2007. "Ethnographic Studies of Childhood: A Historical Overview." *American Anthropologist* 109 (2): 247–260.

Lewis, Charles E., Mary Ann Lewis, Ann Lorimer, and Beverly B. Palmer. 1977. "Child-Initiated Care: The Use of School Nursing Services by Children in an 'Adult-Free' System." *Pediatrics* 60 (4): 499–507.

Liava'a, S. 1998. "Dawn Raids: When Pacific Islanders Were Forced to Go 'Home.'" Master's thesis, University of Auckland.

Littleton, Judith. 2007. "The Production of Local Biologies: Childhood Development at Yuendumu to 1970." *Current Anthropology* 48: 135–45.

Lock, Margaret. 2001. "The Tempering of Medical Anthropology: Troubling Natural Categories." *Medical Anthropology Quarterly* 15: 478–92.

Lundblad, Barbro, and Anna-Lena Hellström. 2005. "Perceptions of School Toilets as a Cause for Irregular Toilet Habits among Schoolchildren Aged 6 to 16 Years." *Journal of School Health* 75 (4): 125–128, https://doi.org/10.1111/j.1746-1561.2005.00009.x.

Luthar, Suniya S., and Dante Cicchetti. 2000. "The Construct of Resilience: Implications for Interventions and Social Policies." *Development and Psychopathology* 12 (4): 857–885.

Macpherson, C. 1996. "Pacific Islands Identity and Community." In *Nga Patai: Racism and Ethnic Relations in Aotearoa/New Zealand*, ed. P. Spoonley, C. Macpherson, and D. Pearson, 124–143. Auckland: Dunmore Press.

Mandell, Nancy. 1988. "The Least-Adult Role in Studying Children." *Journal of Contemporary Ethnography* 16 (4): 433–467.

Mannheim, Karl. 1952. "The Problem of Generations." In *Essays on the Sociology of Knowledge*. London: Routledge & Kegan Paul.

Marie, Dannette, David M. Fergusson, and Joseph M. Boden. 2008. "Educational Achievement in Maori: The Roles of Cultural Identity and Social Disadvantage." *Australian Journal of Education* 52 (2): 183–196, https://doi.org/10.1177/000494410805200206.

Martin, Emily. 1988. "Premenstrual Syndrome: Discipline, Work, and Anger in Late Industrial Societies." In *Blood Magic: The Anthropology of Menstruation*, ed. Thomas Buckley and Alma Gottlieb, 161–181. Berkeley: University of California Press.

———. 1999. "The Woman in the Flexible Body." In *Revisioning Women, Health and Healing: Feminist, Cultural, and Technoscience*, ed. Adele E. Clarke and Virginia L. Olesen, 97–115. New York: Routledge.

Masten, Ann S. 2001. "Ordinary Magic: Resilience Processes in Development." *American Psychologist* 56 (3): 227.

Maton, Karl. 2008. "Habitus." In *Pierre Bourdieu: Key Concepts*, ed. Michael Grenfell, 49–65. Durham, U.K.: Acumen Publishing.

Matthews, Suzanne. 2000. "Reforming Body and Mind: New Zealand Industrial Schools, 1880–1925." In *Public Bodies, Private Lives: A Century of Change in New Zealand Public Health*, ed. Duncan Anderson, 42–56. Hamilton, N.Z.: Social History of Health Group, Department of History, University of Waikato.

Mavoa, Helen. M. 2004. "Mahaki Hela: The Asthma-Related Ideas, Home Interactions and Diurnal Cortisol Patterns of 3–4 Year-Old New Zealand Tongan and Palangi Children with Asthma." Doctoral thesis, University of Auckland.

May, Helen. 2001. "Mapping Some Landscapes of Colonial-global Childhood." *European Early Childhood Education Research Journal* 9 (2): 5–20.

Mayall, Berry. 1993. "Keeping Healthy at Home and School: 'It's My Body, So It's My Job.'" *Sociology of Health & Illness* 15 (4): 464–487.

———. 1994. *Children's Childhoods: Observed and Experienced*. London: Falmer Press.

———. 1996. *Children, Health and the Social Order*. Buckingham PA: Open University Press.

———. 1998. "Towards a Sociology of Child Health." *Sociology of Health & Illness* 20 (3): 269–288.

———. 2000. "Conversations with Children: Working with Generational Issues." In *Research with Children: Perspectives and Practices*, ed. Pia Christensen and Alan Prout, 120–135. London: Falmer Press.

———. 2002. "Children, Emotions and Daily Life at Home and School." In *Emotions in Social Life: Critical Themes and Contemporary Issues*, ed. G. Bendelow and Simon Williams, 135–154. London: Routledge.

———. 2015. "Intergenerational Relations: Embodiment over Time." In *Childhood with Bourdieu*, ed. Leena Alanen, E. Brooker, and Berry Mayall, 13–33. London: Palgrave Macmillan.

McEwen, Bruce S. 1998. "Stress, Adaptation, and Disease: Allostasis and Allostatic Load." *Annals of the New York Academy of Sciences* 840 (1): 33–44.

McIntosh, Caroline M. 2013. "Young Children's Meaning-Making about the Causes of Illness within the Family Context." Doctoral thesis, Massey University.

McIntosh, Tracey. 2001. "Death, Every Day." In *Sociology of Everyday Life in New Zealand*, ed. Claudia Bell, 234–51. Palmerston North, N.Z.: Dunmore Press.

Mead, Margaret. 1930. *Coming of Age in Samoa: A Psychological Study of Primitive Youth for Western Civilization*. New York: Morrow.

Meloni, Francesca, Karine Vanthuyne, and Cécile Rousseau. 2015. "Towards a Relational Ethics: Rethinking Ethics, Agency and Dependency in Research with Children and Youth." *Anthropological Theory* 15 (1): 106–123.

Merleau-Ponty, Maurice. 1962. *Phenomenology of Perception*. New York: Humanities Press.

Meskell, Lynn, and Peter Pels. 2005. "Introduction." In *Embedding Ethics*, ed. Lynn Meskell and Peter Pels, 1–26. Oxford: Berg.

Metge, Joan. 1967. *The Maoris of New Zealand*. Societies of the World. London: Routledge & K. Paul.

———. 1995. *New Growth from Old: The Whānau in the Modern World*. Wellington: Victoria University Press.

Meyer, Roger J., and Robert J. Haggerty. 1962. "Streptoccocal Infections in Families: Factors Altering Individual Susceptibility." *Pediatrics* 29 (4): 539–549.

Migone, Paloma. 2015. "Thousands of Children Hit by Benefit Sanctions." Radio New Zealand, July 24, 2015, https://www.radionz.co.nz/news/national/279597/thousands-of-children-hit-by-benefit-sanctions.

Miller, Peggy J., and Jacqueline J. Goodnow. 1995. "Cultural Practices: Toward an Integration of Culture and Development." *New Directions for Child and Adolescent Development* 1995 (67): 5–16.

Milne, Richard, Diana Lennon, Joanna Stewart, Stephen Vander Hoorn, and Paul Scuffham. 2012. "Incidence of Acute Rheumatic Fever in New Zealand Children and Youth." *Journal of Paediatrics and Child Health* 48 (8): 685–691, https://doi.org/10.1111/j.1440-1754.2012.02447.x.

Ministry of Health. 2012. "The Health of New Zealand Children 2011/12: Key Findings of the New Zealand Health Survey." New Zealand Ministry of Health. Available at http://www.moh.govt.nz/NoteBook/nbbooks.nsf/0/35624B64BEC88496CC257AFA0069BF2A.

———. 2013. "Implementation and Formative Evaluation of the Rheumatic Fever Prevention Programme: Final Report." New Zealand Ministry of Health. Available from http://www.health.govt.nz/our-work/diseases-and-conditions/rheumatic-fever/rheumatic-fever-publications.

———. 2015. "Formative Evaluation of Sore Throat Clinics. Prepared for the Ministry of Health by Litmus Ltd." New Zealand Ministry of Health. Available from http://www.health.govt.nz/our-work/diseases-and-conditions/rheumatic-fever/rheumatic-fever-publications.

———. 2016. "Suicide Facts: Deaths and Intentional Self-Harm Hospitalisations: 2013." New Zealand Ministry of Health. Available from https://www.health.govt.nz/publication/suicide-facts-deaths-and-intentional-self-harm-hospitalisations-2013.

———. 2017. "Previous BPS Target: Reduce Rheumatic Fever." New Zealand Ministry of Health. Available from http://www.health.govt.nz/about-ministry/what-we-do/strategic-direction /better-public-services/previous-bps-target-reduce-rheumatic-fever.

———. 2018. "Reducing Rheumatic Fever." New Zealand Ministry of Health. Available from https://www.health.govt.nz/our-work/diseases-and-conditions/rheumatic-fever /reducing-rheumatic-fever.

Ministry of Social Development. 2012. "The White Paper for Vulnerable Children. Children's Action Plan: Identifying, Supporting and Protecting Vulnerable Children." New Zealand Ministry of Social Development. Available from http://www.childrensactionplan.govt .nz/ the-white-paper.

Mishler, Elliot. 1979. "'Won't You Trade Cookies with the Popcorn': The Talk of Trades among Six Year Olds." In *Language, Children and Society: The Effects of Social Factors on Children's Learning to Communicate*, ed. O. Garnica and M. King, 21–36. Elmsford, NY: Pergamon.

Mitchell, E. A., and D. R. Cutler. 1984. "Paediatric Admissions to Auckland Hospital for Asthma from 1970–1980." *New Zealand Medical Journal* 97 (749): 67–70.

Mizen, Phillip, and Yaw Ofosu-Kusi. 2013. "Agency as Vulnerability: Accounting for Children's Movement to the Streets of Accra." *Sociological Review* 61 (2): 363–382. https:// doi.org/10.1111/1467-954X.12021.

Moir, Jo. 2016. "Government Won't Commit to a Poverty Target Because It's Too 'Difficult'— John Key." *Stuff*, October 13, 2016. Available from https://www.stuff.co.nz/national /politics/84893766/government-wont-commit-to-a-poverty-target-because-its-too -difficult—john-key.

Montgomery, Heather. 2001. *Modern Babylon?: Prostituting Children in Thailand*. New York: Berghahn Books.

———. 2009. *An Introduction to Childhood: Anthropological Perspectives on Children's Lives*. Malden, MA: Wiley-Blackwell.

Moorfield, John C. 2011. *Te Aka: Māori-English, English-Māori Dictionary and Index*. Auckland: Pearson.

Morehu, Colleen. 2005. "A Māori Perspective of Whānau and Childrearing in the 21st Century Case Study." Doctoral thesis, University of Waikato.

Morrison, Marlene. 1996. "Sharing Food at Home and School: Perspectives on Commensality." *Sociological Review* 44 (4): 648–674.

Morton, Helen. 1996. *Becoming Tongan: An Ethnography of Childhood*. Honolulu: University of Hawai'i Press.

Morton, Susan M. B., Polly E. Atatoa Carr, Cameron C. Grant, Elizabeth M. Robinson, Dinusha K. Bandara, Amy Bird, Vivienne C. Ivory, Te Kani R. Kingi, Liang Renee, Emma J. Marks et al. 2013. "Cohort Profile: Growing Up in New Zealand." *International Journal of Epidemiology* 42 (1): 65–75, https://doi.org/10.1093/ije/dyr206.

Muehlenkamp, Jennifer J., Laurence Claes, Lindsey Havertape, and Paul L. Plener. 2012. "International Prevalence of Adolescent Non-Suicidal Self-Injury and Deliberate Self-Harm." *Child and Adolescent Psychiatry and Mental Health* 6 (10): 1–9.

Mutch, Carol Anne, Vivienne Rarere, and Robert Stratford. 2011. "'When You Looked at Me, You Didn't Judge Me': Supporting Transient Students and Their Families in New Zealand Primary Schools." *Pastoral Care in Education* 29 (4): 231–245, https://doi.org/10.1080 /02643944.2011.626065.

Nag, M., B. N. F. White, R. C. Peet, A. Bardhan, T. H. Hull, A. Johnson, G. S. Masnick, S. Polgar, R. Repetto, and S. Tax. 1978. "An Anthropological Approach to the Study of the Economic Value of Children in Java and Nepal [and Comments and Reply]." *Current Anthropology* 19 (2): 293–306.

Nagy, M. H. 1948. "The Child's Theories Concerning Death." *Journal of Genetic Psychology* 73: 3–27.

Nairn, Karen, Jane Higgins, and Judith Sligo. 2012. *Children of Rogernomics: A Neoliberal Generation Leaves School.* Dunedin, N.Z.: Otago University Press.

New Zealand Government. 2018. "Historic Commitment to Reduce Child Poverty." Press release, January 31, 2018. Available from https://beehive.govt.nz/release/historic-commitment-reduce-child-poverty.

New Zealand Herald. 2016. "140,000 Kids Can't Be Wrong." Advertisement. *New Zealand Herald*, August 19, 2016. Available from http://www.nzherald.co.nz/sponsored-stories/news/article.cfm?c_id=1503708&objectid=11696608.

New Zealand Milk Board. 1978. "New Zealand's Milk in Schools Scheme 1937–1967." Wellington: New Zealand Milk Board.

New Zealand National Party. 2018. "National to Support 1st Reading of Child Poverty Legislation." New Zealand National Party press release. *Scoop Independent News*, February 13, 2018, http://www.scoop.co.nz/stories/PA1802/S00105/national-to-support-1st-reading-of-child-poverty-legislation.htm.

Nguyen-Gillham, Viet, Rita Giacaman, Ghada Naser, and Will Boyce. 2008. "Normalizing the Abnormal: Palestinian Youth and the Contradictions of Resilience in Protracted Conflict." *Health & Social Care in the Community* 16 (3): 291–298.

Nichter, Mark. 2003. "Harm Reduction: A Core Concern for Medical Anthropology." In *Risk, Culture, and Health Inequality: Shifting Perceptions of Danger and Blame*, ed. Barbara Herr Harthorn and Laury Oaks, 13–33. Westport, CT: Praeger.

Nieuwenhuys, O. 1996. "The Paradox of Child Labor and Anthropology." *Annual Review of Anthropology* 25: 237–251.

Nikula, Pii-Tuulia. 2018. "Let's Look to Finland and Adopt Universal Free School Lunches." *Stuff*, February 9, 2018. Available from http://www.stuff.co.nz/national/education/101305452/lets-look-to-finland-and-adopt-universal-free-school-lunches.

O'Brien, Michael. 2016. "The Triplets: Investment in Outcomes for the Vulnerable—Reshaping Social Services for (Some) New Zealand Children." *Aotearoa New Zealand Social Work Review* 28 (2): 9–21, https://doi.org/doi:10.11157/anzswj-vol28iss2id220.

Ochs, Elinor. 1993. "Constructing Social Identity: A Language Socialization Perspective." *Research on Language and Social Interaction* 26 (3): 287–306.

Oliver, Melody, Elaine Rush, Philip Schluter, Gerhard Sundborn, Leon Iusitini, El-Shadan Tautolo, Janis Paterson, and James Heimuli. 2011. "An Exploration of Physical Activity, Nutrition, and Body Size in Pacific Children." *Pacific Health Dialog* 17 (2): 176–196.

Opie, Iona Archibald, and Peter Opie. 1969. *Children's Games.* Oxford: Oxford University Press.

Orellana, Marjorie F. 2009. *Translating Childhoods: Immigrant Youth, Language, and Culture.* New Brunswick, NJ: Rutgers University Press.

Ortner, Sherry B. 1984. "Theory in Anthropology since the Sixties." *Comparative Studies in Society and History* 26 (1): 126–166.

———. 2006. *Anthropology and Social Theory: Culture, Power, and the Acting Subject.* Durham, NC: Duke University Press.

Penehira, Mera, Alison Green, Linda Tuhiwai Smith, and Clive Aspin. 2014. "Māori and Indigenous Views on R and R: Resistance and Resilience." *Mai Journal* 3 (2): 96–110.

Panter-Brick, Catherine. 1998a. "Biological Anthropology and Child Health: Context, Process and Outcome." In *Biosocial Perspectives on Children*, ed. Catherine Panter-Brick, 66–101. Cambridge: Cambridge University Press.

———. 1998b. *Biosocial Perspectives on Children.* Cambridge: Cambridge University Press.

———. 2002. "Street Children, Human Rights, and Public Health: A Critique and Future Directions." *Annual Review of Anthropology* 31: 147–171.

Panter-Brick, Catherine, and Mark Eggerman. 2012. "Understanding Culture, Resilience, and Mental Health: The Production of Hope." In *The Social Ecology of Resilience: A Handbook of Theory and Practice*, ed. Michael Ungar, 369–386. New York: Springer.

Panter-Brick, Catherine, Mark Eggerman, V. Gonzalez, and S. Safdar. 2009. "Violence, Suffering, and Mental Health in Afghanistan: A School-Based Survey." *Lancet* 374: 807–16.

Panter-Brick, Catherine, Anna Goodman, Wietse Tol, and Mark Eggerman. 2011. "Mental Health and Childhood Adversities: A Longitudinal Study in Kabul, Afghanistan." *Journal of the American Academy of Child & Adolescent Psychiatry* 50 (4): 349–363.

Panter-Brick, Catherine, and James F. Leckman. 2013. "Editorial Commentary: Resilience in Child Development–interconnected Pathways to Wellbeing." *Journal of Child Psychology and Psychiatry* 54 (4): 333–336.

Panter-Brick, Catherine, and T. M. Pollard. 1999. "Work and Hormonal Variation in Subsistence and Industrial Contexts." In *Hormones, Health, and Behavior*, ed. Catherine Panter-Brick and Carol. M. Worthman, 139–183. Cambridge: Cambridge University Press.

Panter-Brick, Catherine, Linda C. Theron, Linda Liebenberg, and Michael Ungar. 2015. "Culture and Resilience: Next Steps for Theory and Practice." In *Youth Resilience and Culture. Cross-Cultural Advancements in Positive Psychology*, 233–244. New York: Springer.

Panter-Brick, Catherine, A. Todd, and R. Baker. 1996. "Growth Status of Homeless Nepali Boys: Do They Differ from Rural and Urban Controls?" *Social Science & Medicine* 43: 441–451.

Park, Julie. 2000. "'The Worst Hassle Is You Can't Play Rugby': Haemophilia and Masculinity in New Zealand." *Current Anthropology* 41 (3): 444–453, https://doi.org/10.1086/300151.

Parsons, Ross. 2012. *One Day This Will All Be Over: Growing up with HIV in Eastern Zimbabwe*. Harare, Zimbabwe: Weaver Press.

Parsons, Talcott. 1951. *The Social System*. London: Routledge and Kegan Paul.

Patterson, Jane. 2017. "Minor Parties Wade into Child Poverty Debate." Radio New Zealand, September 5, 2017. Available from https://www.radionz.co.nz/news/political/338739/minor-parties-wade-into-child-poverty-debate.

Pearce, Jamie, and Danny Dorling. 2006. "Increasing Geographical Inequalities in Health in New Zealand, 1980–2001." *International Journal of Epidemiology* 35 (3): 597–603. https://doi.org/10.1093/ije/dyl013.

Pels, Peter. 2005. "'Where There Aren't No Ten Commandments': Redefining Ethics During the Darkness in El Dorado Scandal." In *Embedding Ethics*, ed. Lynn Meskell and Peter Pels, 69–100. Oxford: Berg.

Pennebaker, James W. 1982. *The Psychology of Physical Symptoms*. New York: Springer-Verlag.

———. 2000. "Psychological Factors Influencing the Reporting of Physical Symptoms." In *The Science of Self-Report: Implications for Research and Practice*, ed. Arthur A. Stone, Christine A. Bachrach, Jared B. Jobe, Howard S. Kutzman, and Virginia S. Cain, 299–315. Mahwah, NJ: Lawrence Erlbaum.

Perry, B. 2016. "Household Incomes in New Zealand, Trends in Indicators of Inequality and Hardship 1982 to 2014." New Zealand Ministry of Social Development. Available from http:// www.msd.govt.nz/about-msd-and-our-work/publications-resources/monitoring/householdincomes/.

Peters, Michael A., and Tina Besley. 2014. "Children in Crisis: Child Poverty and Abuse in New Zealand." *Educational Philosophy and Theory* 46 (9): 945–961, https://doi.org/10.1080/00131857.2014.935280.

PHARMAC. n.d. "One Heart Many Lives." OHML. Accessed 23 March 2017. Available from http://www.oneheartmanylives.co.nz/.

Piaget, Jean. 1967. *Six Psychological Studies*. New York: Random House.

Pihama, Leonie, Paul Reynolds, Cherryl Smith, John Reid, Linda Tuhiwai Smith, and Rihi Te Nana. 2014. "Positioning Historical Trauma Theory within Aotearoa New Zealand." *AlterNative: An International Journal of Indigenous Peoples* 10 (3): 248–262.

Pink, Sarah. 2013. *Doing Visual Ethnography*. 3rd edition. Los Angeles, CA: Sage.

Poata-Smith, Evan Te Ahu. 2013. "Inequality and Māori." In *Inequality: A New Zealand Crisis*, ed. Max Rashbrooke, 148–158. Wellington: Bridget Williams Books.

Poulton, Richie, Avshalom Caspi, Barry J. Milne, W. Murray Thomson, Alan Taylor, Malcolm R. Sears, and Terrie E. Moffitt. 2002. "Association between Children's Experience of Socioeconomic Disadvantage and Adult Health: A Life-Course Study." *Lancet* 360 (9346): 1640–1645, https://doi.org/10.1016/S0140-6736(02)11602-3.

Poulton, Richie, Terrie E. Moffitt, and Phil A. Silva. 2015. "The Dunedin Multidisciplinary Health and Development Study: Overview of the First 40 Years, with an Eye to the Future." *Social Psychiatry and Psychiatric Epidemiology* 50 (5): 679–693, https://doi.org/10.1007/s00127-015-1048-8.

Prendergast, Shirley. 2000. "'To Become Dizzy in Our Turning': Girls, Body-Maps and Gender as Childhood Ends." In *The Body, Childhood and Society*, ed. Alan Prout. London: Palgrave Macmillan.

Prendergast, Shirley, and S. Forrest. 1998. "'Shorties, Low-Lifers, Hard Nuts and Kings': Boys and the Transformation of Emotions." In *Emotions in Social Life: Social Theories and Contemporary Issues*, ed. G. Bendelow and Simon Williams. London: Routledge.

Price, David H. 2016. "Be Open and Honest Regarding Your Work." In *Anthropological Ethics in Context: An Ongoing Dialogue*, ed. Dena Plemmons and Alex W. Barker, 91–106. Walnut Creek, CA: Left Coast Press.

Prout, Alan. 1986. "'Wet Children' and 'Little Actresses': Going Sick in Primary School." *Sociology of Health & Illness* 8 (2): 113–136.

———. 2000a. "Childhood Bodies: Construction, Agency and Hybridity." In *The Body, Childhood and Society*, ed. Alan Prout, 1–18. London: Palgrave Macmillan.

———. ed. 2000b. *The Body, Childhood and Society*. London: Palgrave Macmillan.

———. 2005. *The Future of Childhood: Towards the Interdisciplinary Study of Children*. London: Routledge Falmer.

Prout, Alan, and Pia Christensen. 1996. "Hierarchies, Boundaries, and Symbols: Medicine Use and the Cultural Performance of Childhood Sickness." In *Children, Medicines, and Culture*, ed. Patricia Bush, Deanna Trakas, Emilio J. Sanz, Rolf L. Wirsing, Tuula Vaskilampi, and Alan Prout, 31–54. London: Pharmaceutical Press.

Quesada, James, Laurie Kain Hart, and Philippe Bourgois. 2011. "Structural Vulnerability and Health: Latino Migrant Laborers in the United States." *Medical Anthropology* 30 (4): 339–362, https://doi.org/10.1080/01459740.2011.576725.

Qvortrup, Jens. 1994. "Introduction." In *Childhood Matters: Social Theory, Practice, and Politics*, ed. Jens Qvortrup, Marjatta Bardy, Giovanni Sgritta, and Helmut Wintersbergery. Aldershot, Hampshire, U.K.: Avebury.

Radio New Zealand. 2017. "English Pledges to Lift 100k Children out of Poverty." Radio New Zealand, September 5, 2017. Available from https://www.radionz.co.nz/national/programmes/morningreport/audio/201857293/english-pledges-to-lift-100k-children-out-of-poverty.

Ramos, Manuel João. 2004. "Drawing the Lines: The Limitations of Intercultural Ekphrasis." In *Working Images: Visual Research and Representation in Ethnography*, edited by Sarah Pink, László Kürti, and Ana Isabel Afonso. London; New York: Routledge.

Ramsay, Samantha A., Laurel J. Branen, Janice Fletcher, Elizabeth Price, Susan L. Johnson, and Madeleine Sigman-Grant. 2010. "'Are You Done?' Child Care Providers' Verbal Communication at Mealtimes That Reinforce or Hinder Children's Internal Cues of Hunger and Satiation." *Journal of Nutrition Education and Behavior* 42 (4): 265–270.

Randall, Duncan. 2012. "Revisiting Mandell's 'Least Adult' Role and Engaging with Children's Voices in Research." *Nurse Researcher* 19 (3): 39–43.

Rashbrooke, Max. 2013. *Inequality: A New Zealand Crisis*. Wellington: Bridget Williams Books.

———. 2017. "Surprise! National Can Measure Child Poverty after All. Now Comes the Hard Part." *Spinoff*, September 5, 2017. Available from https://thespinoff.co.nz/politics/05-09-2017/surprise-national-can-measure-child-poverty-after-all-now-comes-the-hard-part/.

Read, M. 1968. *Children of Their Fathers: Growing Up among the Ngoni of Malawi*. New York: Holt, Rinehart & Winston.

Reid, John, Karyn Taylor-Moore, and Golda Varona. 2014. "Towards a Social-Structural Model for Understanding Current Disparities in Maori Health and Well-Being." *Journal of Loss and Trauma* 19 (6): 514–536.

Reid, John, Golda Varona, Martin Fisher, and Cherryl Smith. 2016. "Understanding Maori 'Lived' Culture to Determine Cultural Connectedness and Wellbeing." *Journal of Population Research* 33 (1): 31–49, https://doi.org/10.1007/s12546-016-9165-0.

Reynolds, Pamela. 1991. *Dance, Civet Cat: Child Labour in the Zambezi Valley*. London: Baobab Books.

Rice, G. 1996. "A Revolution in Social Policy, 1981–1991." In *The Oxford History of New Zealand*, 2nd ed., ed. G. Rice, 482–497. Auckland: Oxford University Press.

Ritchie, Jane. 1957. *Childhood in Rakau: The First Five Years of Life*. Wellington: Department of Psychology, Victoria University College.

Ritchie, Jane, and James E. Ritchie. 1970. *Child Rearing Patterns in New Zealand*. Wellington: AH & AW Reed.

———. 1979. *Growing Up in Polynesia*. Sydney: Allen & Unwin.

———. 1997. *The Next Generation: Child Rearing in New Zealand*. Auckland: Penguin.

Roberts, R. L., T. R. Merriman, and J. D. Upton. 2010. "Letters to the Editors: High Frequency of MCM6 Lactose Intolerance Genotype in Polynesian People." *Alimentary Pharmacology & Therapeutics* 32 (6): 828–829, https://doi.org/10.1111/j.1365-2036.2010.04398.x.

Robin, Audrey, Clair Mills, Roger Tuck, and Diana R. Lennon. 2013. "The Epidemiology of Acute Rheumatic Fever in Northland, 2002–2011." *New Zealand Medical Journal* (online) 126 (1373).

Robson, Elsbeth. 2004. "Hidden Child Workers: Young Carers in Zimbabwe." *Antipode* 36 (2): 227–248.

Rose, Nikolas. 1999. *Governing the Soul: The Shaping of the Private Self*. London: Routledge.

———. 2007. *Politics of Life Itself: Biomedicine, Power, and Subjectivity in the Twenty-First Century*. Princeton, NJ: Princeton University Press.

Rosenblatt, Daniel. 2011. "Indigenizing the City and the Future of Maori Culture: The Construction of Community in Auckland as Representation, Experience, and Self-Making." *American Ethnologist* 38 (3): 411–429.

Rozin, Paul, Sara Dow, Morris Moscovitch, and Suparna Rajaram. 1998. "What Causes Humans to Begin and End a Meal? A Role for Memory for What Has Been Eaten, as

Evidenced by a Study of Multiple Meal Eating in Amnesic Patients." *Psychological Science* 9 (5): 392–396.

Rutter, Michael. 1987. "Psychosocial Resilience and Protective Mechanisms." *American Journal of Orthopsychiatry* 57 (3): 316.

———. 2013. "Annual Research Review: Resilience—Clinical Implications." *Journal of Child Psychology and Psychiatry* 54 (4): 474–487.

Ryan, Kevin William. 2012. "The New Wave of Childhood Studies: Breaking the Grip of Bio-Social Dualism?" *Childhood* 19 (4): 439–452.

Sahlins, Marshall. 1981. *Historical Metaphors and Mythical Realities: Structure in the Early History of the Sandwich Islands Kingdom.* Ann Arbor: University of Michigan Press.

Salmond, Anne. 1976. *Hui: A Study of Maori Ceremonial Gatherings.* Auckland: Reed Methuen.

Saunders, J. Llewellyn. 1964. *The New Zealand School Dental Service: Its Initiation and Development 1920–1960.* Wellington: Government Printing Office.

Savelio, A. 2005. "'Shut the Door—They're Coming Through the Window': An Immigration and Citizenship Crisis Between the New Zealand Government and the People of Samoa, in 1982." Master's thesis, University of Auckland.

Savila, Mr Fa'asisila, G. Sundborn, A. Hirao, and J. Paterson. 2011. "Ten Years of Research for the Pacific Islands Families Study: A Comparative Review of Publications." *Pacific Dialogue* 17 (2): 188.

Scheper-Hughes, Nancy. 1993. *Death without Weeping: The Violence of Everyday Life in Brazil.* Berkeley: University of California Press.

———. 1995. "The Primacy of the Ethical: Propositions for a Militant Anthropology." *Current Anthropology* 36 (3): 409–440.

———. 1996. "Small Wars and Invisible Genocides." *Social Science & Medicine* (XIVth International Conference on the Social Sciences and Medicine), 43 (5): 889–900, https://doi.org/10.1016/0277-9536(96)00152-9.

———. 2004. "Dangerous and Endangered Youth: Social Structures and Determinants of Violence." *Annals of the New York Academy of Sciences* 1036 (1): 13–46.

———. 2008. "A Talent for Life: Reflections on Human Vulnerability and Resilience." *Ethnos* 73 (1): 25–56.

Schieffelin, Bambi B. 1990. *The Give and Take of Everyday Life: Language, Socialization of Kaluli Children.* Cambridge: Cambridge University Press.

Schieffelin, Bambi B., and Elinor Ochs. 1986. "Language Socialization." *Annual Review of Anthropology* 15 (1): 163–191.

Schwartzman, Helen B. 2001. "Children and Anthropology: A Century of Studies." In *Children and Anthropology. Perspectives for the 21st Century,* ed. Helen B. Schwartzman, 15–37. Westport, CT: Bergin & Garvey.

Scott, Kathryn, Patricia Laing, and Julie Park. 2016. *Housing Children: South Auckland—The Housing Pathways Longitudinal Study.* Research in Anthropology and Linguistics Electronic Series No. 6, University of Auckland, Department of Anthropology. Available from https://cdn.auckland.ac.nz/assets/arts/schools/anthropology/rale-06.pdf.

Shilling, Chris. 1993. *The Body and Social Theory.* London: Sage.

Shore, Cris. 2017. "Audit Culture and the Politics of Responsibility: Beyond Neoliberal Responsibilization?" In *Competing Responsibilities: The Ethics and Politics of Contemporary Life,* ed. Susanna Trnka and Catherine Trundle, 96–117. Durham, NC: Duke University Press.

Shore, Cris, and Susanna Trnka. 2013. "Introduction—Observing Anthropologists: Professional Knowledge, Practice and Lives." In *Up Close and Personal: On Peripheral Perspectives and the Production of Anthropological Knowledge,* ed. Cris Shore and Susanna Trnka, 1–33. New York: Berghahn Books.

Silva, Phil A. 1990. "The Dunedin Multidisciplinary Health and Development Study: A 15 Year Longitudinal Study." *Paediatric and Perinatal Epidemiology* 4 (1): 76–107, https://doi .org/10.1111/j.1365-3016.1990.tb00621.x.

Sinclair, Karen. 1990. "Tangi: Funeral Rituals and the Construction of Maori Identity." In *Cultural Identity and Ethnicity in the Pacific*, ed. Jocelyn Linnekin and Lin Poyer, 169–73. Honolulu: University of Hawai'i Press.

Sinclair, Keith. 2000. *A History of New Zealand*, rev. ed. Auckland: Penguin Books.

Sinkinson, Margaret. 2011. "Back to the Future: Reoccurring Issues and Discourses in Health Education in New Zealand Schools." *Policy Futures in Education* 9 (3): 315–27. https://doi.org/10.2304/pfie.2011.9.3.315.

Smart, Carol. 2007. *Personal Life*. Cambridge: Polity.

Smith, Anne B. 2013. *Understanding Children and Childhood: A New Zealand Perspective*. Wellington: Bridget Williams Books.

Smith, Michelle Ann. 2016. *Open All Hours: Main Street Papakura c.1865–1938*. Auckland: Papakura and Districts Historical Society and Papakura Museum.

Social Security Act 1964. No. 136. Available from http://www.legislation.govt.nz/act/public/1964/0136/latest/whole.html.

Spray, Julie, Bruce Floyd, Judith Littleton, Susanna Trnka, and Siobhan Mattison. 2018. "Social Group Dynamics Predict Stress Variability among Children in a New Zealand Classroom." *HOMO* 69 (1–2): 50–61.

Stack, Carol. 1974. *All Our Kin*. New York, NY: Basic Books.

Statistics New Zealand. 2015. "New Zealand Period Life Tables: 2012–14." Available from http://www.stats.govt.nz/browse_for_stats/health/life_expectancy/NZLifeTables_ HOTP12-14.aspx.

Steele, B. T. 1973. "Measles in Auckland 1971–1972." *New Zealand Medical Journal* 77: 293–297.

Steggals, Peter. 2015. *Making Sense of Self-Harm: The Cultural Meaning and Social Context of Nonsuicidal Self-Injury*. London: Palgrave Macmillan.

Stephens, Sharon, ed. 1995. *Children and the Politics of Culture*. Princeton, NJ: Princeton University Press.

Tap, Relinde. 2007. "High-Wire Dancers: Middle-Class Pakeha and Dutch Childhoods in New Zealand." Doctoral thesis, University of Auckland.

Taxation (Working for Families) Act 2004, No. 52. Available from http://www.legislation. govt.nz/act/public/2004/0052/latest/DLM299520.html.

Telfar-Barnard, Lucy, Nick Preval, Philippa Howden-Chapman, Richard Arnold, Chris Young, Arthur Grimes, and Tim Denne. 2011. "The Impact of Retrofitted Insulation and New Heaters on Health Services Utilisation and Costs, Pharmaceutical Costs and Mortality: Evaluation of Warm Up New Zealand: Heat Smart." University of Otago at Wellington. Available from http://www.healthyhousing.org.nz/wp-content/uploads/2012/03/ NZIF_Health_report-Final.pdf.

The Open University. n.d. "Children's Research Centre." Accessed March 14, 2018, from http://www.open.ac.uk/researchprojects/childrens-research-centre/.

Theron, Linda C., and Adam M. C. Theron. 2011. "Culturally Embedded Meaning Making: An Exploration of How Young Resilient South African Adults Confront Suffering." In paper accepted for the Second International Making Sense of Suffering Conference, Prague, 9–11. Available from http://www.inter-disciplinary.net/wp-content/uploads /2011/10/theronsufpaper.pdf.

Thomson, Patricia. 2008. "Field." In *Pierre Bourdieu: Key Concepts*, ed. Michael Grenfell, 67–81. Durham, U.K.: Acumen Publishing.

Thorne, Barrie. 1993. *Gender Play: Girls and Boys in School*. New Brunswick, N.J.: Rutgers University Press.
———. 2007. "Editorial: Crafting the Interdisciplinary Field of Childhood Studies." *Childhood* 14 (2): 147–152.
Thorns, D. 2000. "Housing Policy in the 1990s—New Zealand a Decade of Change." *Housing Studies* 15 (1): 129–138.
Toren, Christina. 1990. *Making Sense of Hierarchy: Cognition as Social Process in Fiji*. Monographs on Social Anthropology, No. 61. Atlantic Highlands, NJ: Athlone Press.
———. 1993. "Making History: The Significance of Childhood Cognition for a Comparative Anthropology of Mind." *Man* 28 (3): 461–478, https://doi.org/10.2307/2804235.
———. 1999. *Mind, Materiality, and History: Essays in Fijian Ethnography*. New York: Routledge.
Trnka, Susanna. 2017. *One Blue Child: Asthma, Personal Responsibility, and the Politics of 21st Century Patienthood*. Stanford, CA: Stanford University Pres.
Trnka, Susanna, and Catherine Trundle. 2017. "Competing Responsibilities: Reckoning Personal Responsibility, Care for the Other, and the Social Contract in Contemporary Life." In *Competing Responsibilities: The Ethics and Politics of Contemporary Life*, ed. Susanna Trnka and Catherine Trundle, 1–24. Durham, NC: Duke University Press.
Turner, Bryan S. 1984. *The Body and Society*. Oxford: Blackwell
———. 1992. *Regulating Bodies: Essays in Medical Sociology*. London: Routledge
Turner, Hana, Christine M. Rubie-Davies, and Melinda Webber. 2015. "Teacher Expectations, Ethnicity and the Achievement Gap." *New Zealand Journal of Educational Studies* 50 (1): 55–69.
Ungar, Michael. 2011. "The Social Ecology of Resilience: Addressing Contextual and Cultural Ambiguity of a Nascent Construct." *American Journal of Orthopsychiatry* 81: 1–17.
———. 2012. "Social Ecologies and Their Contribution to Resilience." In *The Social Ecology of Resilience: A Handbook of Theory and Practice*, ed. Michael Ungar, 13–31. New York: Springer.
Ungar, Michael, Marion Brown, Linda Liebenberg, Maria Cheung, and Kathryn Levine. 2008. "Distinguishing Differences in Pathways to Resilience among Canadian Youth." *Canadian Journal of Community Mental Health* 27 (1): 1–13.
Ungar, Michael, Marion Brown, Linda Liebenberg, and Rasha Othman. 2007. "Unique Pathways to Resilience across Cultures." *Adolescence* 42 (166): 287.
Ungar, Michael, Mehdi Ghazinour, and Jörg Richter. 2013. "Annual Research Review: What Is Resilience within the Social Ecology of Human Development?" *Journal of Child Psychology and Psychiatry* 54 (4): 348–366.
UNICEF Office of Research. 2017. "Building the Future: Children and the Sustainable Development Goals in Rich Countries." Innocenti Report Card 14. Florence: UNICEF Office of Research.
United Nations. 2015. "Transforming Our World: The 2030 Agenda for Sustainable Development." Available from https://sustainabledevelopment.un.org/post2015/transforming ourworld.
Utter, Jennifer, Robert Scragg, Cliona Ni Mhurchu, and David Schaaf. 2007. "At-Home Breakfast Consumption among New Zealand Children: Associations with Body Mass Index and Related Nutrition Behaviors." *Journal of the American Dietetic Association* 107 (4): 570–576.
Valentine, Gill. 2009. "Children's Bodies: An Absent Presence." In *Contested Bodies of Childhood and Youth*, ed. Kathrin Hörschelmann and Rachel Colls, 22–37. London: Palgrave Macmillan.

van Meijl, T.. 2006. "Multiple Identifications and the Dialogical Self: Urban Maori Youngsters and the Cultural Renaissance." *Journal of the Royal Anthropological Institute* 12 (4).

Veasy, L. George, Susan E. Wiedmeier, Garth S. Orsmond, Herbert D. Ruttenberg, Mark M. Boucek, Stephen J. Roth, Vera F. Tait, Joel A. Thompson, Judy A. Daly, and Edward L. Kaplan. 1987. "Resurgence of Acute Rheumatic Fever in the Intermountain Area of the United States." *New England Journal of Medicine* 316 (8): 421–427.

Vermillion Peirce, P., S. Akroyd, and P. Tafuna. 2015. "Evaluation of the 2015 Rheumatic Fever Awareness Campaign." New Zealand Ministry of Health. Available from http://www.health.govt.nz/publication/evaluation-2015-rheumatic-fever-awareness-campaign.

Vuorisalo, Mari, and Leena Alanen. 2015. "Early Childhood Education as a Social Field: Everyday Struggles and Practices of Dominance." In *Childhood with Bourdieu*, edited by Leena Alanen, E. Brooker, and Berry Mayall, 78–98. New York, NY: Palgrave McMillan.

Vygotsky, L.S. 1978. *Mind in Society: The Development of Higher of Psychological Processes.* Cambridge, MA: Harvard University Press.

Wacquant, Loïc. 2004. *Body & Soul: Notebooks of an Apprentice Boxer.* Oxford: Oxford University Press Oxford.

———. 2005. "Habitus." In *International Encyclopedia of Economic Sociology*, ed. J. Becket and Z. Milan, 317–321. London: Routledge.

———. 2016. "A Concise Genealogy and Anatomy of Habitus." *Sociological Review* 64 (1): 64–72.

Waksler, Frances Chaput. 1986. "Studying Children: Phenomenological Insights." *Human Studies* 9 (1): 71–82.

Walters, Karina L., Selina A. Mohammed, Teresa Evans-Campbell, Ramona E. Beltrán, David H. Chae, and Bonnie Duran. 2011. "Bodies Don't Just Tell Stories, They Tell Histories: Embodiment of Historical Trauma among American Indians and Alaska Natives." *Du Bois Review: Social Science Research on Race* 8 (1): 179–189.

Wang, Xiying, and Petula Sik Ying Ho. 2007. "My Sassy Girl: A Qualitative Study of Women's Aggression in Dating Relationships in Beijing." *Journal of Interpersonal Violence* 22 (5): 623–638.

Wansink, Brian, James E. Painter, and Jill North. 2005. "Bottomless Bowls: Why Visual Cues of Portion Size May Influence Intake." *Obesity Research* 13 (1): 93–100.

Wham, C. A., R. Teh, S. Moyes, L. Dyall, M. Kepa, K. Hayman, and N. Kerse. 2015. "Health and Social Factors Associated with Nutrition Risk: Results from Life and Living in Advanced Age: A Cohort Study in New Zealand (LILACS NZ)." *Journal of Nutrition, Health & Aging* 19 (6): 637–645.

Wiley, Andrea S. 2007. "The Globalization of Cow's Milk Production and Consumption: Biocultural Perspectives." *Ecology of Food and Nutrition* 46 (3–4): 281–312.

———. 2014. *Cultures of Milk: The Biology and Meaning of Dairy Products in the United States and India.* Cambridge, MA: Harvard University Press.

Wilkinson, Paul, and Ian Goodyer. 2011. "Non-Suicidal Self-Injury." *European Child & Adolescent Psychiatry* 20 (2): 103–108.

Wilson, C., C. C. Grant, and C. R. Wall. 1999. "Iron Deficiency Anaemia and Adverse Dietary Habits in Hospitalised Children." *New Zealand Medical Journal* 112: 203–206.

Wilson, Nigel J. 2010. "Rheumatic Heart Disease in Indigenous Populations—New Zealand Experience." *Heart, Lung and Circulation* 19 (5): 282–288.

Wilson, Nigel J., M. Baker, D. Martin, Diana R. Lennon, J. O'Hallahan, N. Jones, J. Wenger, O. Mansoor, M. Thomas, and C. Jefferies. 1995. "Meningococcal Disease Epidemiology and Control in New Zealand." *New Zealand Medical Journal* 108 (1010): 437–442.

Wirihana, Rebecca, and Cherryl Smith. 2014. "Historical Trauma, Healing and Well-Being in Maori Communities." *Mai Journal* 3 (3): 197–210.

Worthman, C. M. 1993. "Biocultural Interactions in Human Development." In *Juvenile Primates: Life History, Development, and Behavior*, ed. M. E. Pereira and L. A. Fairbanks, 339–358. New York: Oxford University Press.

Wrong, Dennis H. 1961. "The Oversocialized Conception of Man in Modern Sociology." *American Sociological Review*, 26(2): 183–193.

Wynd, Donna. 2014. *The Revolving Door: Student Mobility in Auckland Schools*. Auckland: Child Poverty Action Group.

Yehuda, Rachel, and Janine D. Flory. 2007. "Differentiating Biological Correlates of Risk, PTSD, and Resilience Following Trauma Exposure." *Journal of Traumatic Stress* 20 (4): 435–447.

Young, Allan. 1982. "The Anthropologies of Illness and Sickness." *Annual Review of Anthropology* 11 (1): 257–285.

Young, Audrey. 2015. "Government Votes Down 'Feed the Kids' Bill." *New Zealand Herald*, March 19, 2015. Available from http://www.nzherald.co.nz/nz/news/article.cfm?c_id=1&objectid=11419393.

INDEX

abuse: child, 33, 44, 63, 160, 204n4, 204n7; peer, 148
accommodations, for resilience, 141–142, 145, 155–156, 162–163, 190
adolescence, adolescents: care for, 109, 111, 113; cultural meanings of, 18; resilience of, 143–144, 151, 155, 158; and risk, 159, 162, 170, 185
adoption. *See* whāngai
adult: authority, power, 13, 46–54, 60, 65, 89, 118, 156–158, 169–170; difference from children, 175–176, 178; growing into, 10, 16, 18–19, 84, 107, 116–117, 120, 154, 166; influence on children, 7–8, 16, 43, 124–125, 128, 154; roles in care, 76–78, 89–90, 93–98, 110–112, 137, 170–171; roles in research, 48–66, 121. *See also* adult-centrism; adulthood
adult-centrism: agendas, 68; assumptions, 3, 76, 130, 145–147; expectations of children, 6, 48, 57, 60, 165–166; misrecognition of children, 160–162, 180–183; normative values, 143, 155; of social structures, 49, 169–171, 188–193
adulthood, children's perspectives of, 1, 52, 96–97, 111
adversity, 8, 33, 140, 142–143, 151, 156
advertising. *See* health promotion
affect, affection, 45, 94, 96, 98, 192, 197
agency, children's: in biosocial processes, 115, 117; and care, 93, 95, 98; in coproduction, 17, 19, 90, 190; in illness, 3, 8, 93; in research processes, 65; in resilience, 140, 142–146, 150, 151, 154, 162–163; and socialization, 10–11; theories of, 8–11, 16. *See also* structure-agency tension
aggression, 130–132, 142, 151, 154–158, 162–163, 190
anthropology: biological, 9, 17–19, 115–117, 156; of childhood, 7–11, 17–19, 43–44, 47, 53, 67, 93, 114–116
antibiotics: children's use of, 3, 5, 39, 82–86, 90, 146, 181; in RF prevention, 38–39, 70–71, 108–110, 184–186; social meanings of, 82–86, 88, 146; understandings of, 54. *See also* pharmaceuticals
anxiety, 76, 84, 86, 109, 134, 137, 162, 180–181, 205n5

Aotearoa (New Zealand): anthropology of, 7, 43; constructions of childhood, 18, 24, 30, 170–171; cultural features, 32, 43–44, 122, 124; ethnic groups, 24–27, 34–38; history of, 1, 24–25, 34–36, 41–42, 98, 105; inequities within, 24–25, 31–39, 43–44, 187; law, 24, 44, 63–64, 155, 170; politics of, 91, 93, 98–99, 112, 187–188. *See also* policy
asthma, 2–3, 6, 37, 88, 123, 134–135
attunement, 21, 118–120, 124–125, 127, 133, 136–137, 186
Auckland, 1, 5, 24–26, 34–37, 43, 122, 165, 186
authority: adult, 16, 46–51, 53–54, 61–62, 65–68, 77, 87, 89, 111, 125, 161, 197; institutional, 46–47, 67–68 118, 161; medical, 77, 79, 82, 98
autonomy, 65, 98, 111, 116, 118, 151, 154, 163, 178. *See also* agency

bacteria, Group A Streptococcus (GAS), 38–39, 70, 86, 130, 146, 182
bathrooms, toilets, 46, 58–61, 118. *See also* toileting
behavior: as expression, 175; health behaviors, 4, 41, 190; in peer cultures, 55–60, 150, 155, 159–163; of researcher, 49, 52, 55–63; responses to distress, 155–163, 176–177; socially produced, 15, 18, 94, 115–118, 150; unsanctioned, taboo, 27, 48, 55–60, 155–162, 206n7
biocultural, biosocial processes, 4, 8–10, 16, 18–19, 115–120, 127–128, 137–138
Bluebond-Langner, Myra, 6–7, 165–166, 175
body: coproduction of, 5, 8–10, 17, 20, 68, 72–73, 137–138, 190–191; experience of, 2–5, 17, 72, 76–80, 123–127, 133–137, 170, 177–178, 189, 197; incarnate and somatic, 17, 77–79, 83–84, 191; and power, 46, 57; practices of, 142, 154–155, 157–160, 163, 178; socialized, 128–129, 133–134; theories of, 4, 9–10, 17–19, 67, 114–121, 127–128; understandings of, 76–89; variation of, 100; weight, 100, 110–111, 205n3. *See also* embodiment
boundaries, 6, 46, 197

231

ABOUT THE AUTHOR

With a background in both biological and social anthropology, JULIE SPRAY brings unique interdisciplinary approaches to her research with New Zealand children. Her academic work focuses on developing creative ways of examining issues related to child health and well-being. She holds doctoral and master's degrees from the University of Auckland. She also holds an honors degree in fine arts from the University of Auckland, which has influenced her visual anthropology practice—including many of the illustrations in this book.

Available titles in the Rutgers Series in Childhood Studies:

Edward W. Morris, *Learning the Hard Way: Masculinity, Place, and the Gender Gap in Education*

Erin N. Winkler, *Learning Race, Learning Place: Shaping Racial Identities and Ideas in African American Childhoods*

Jenny Huberman, *Ambivalent Encounters: Childhood, Tourism, and Social Change in Banaras, India*

Walter Hamilton, *Children of the Occupation: Japan's Untold Story*

Jon M. Wolseth, *Life on the Malecón: Children and Youth on the Streets of Santo Domingo*

Lisa M. Nunn, *Defining Student Success: The Role of School and Culture*

Vikki S. Katz, *Kids in the Middle: How Children of Immigrants Negotiate Community Interactions for Their Families*

Bambi L. Chapin, *Childhood in a Sri Lankan Village: Shaping Hierarchy and Desire*

David M. Rosen, *Child Soldiers in the Western Imagination: From Patriots to Victims*

Marianne Modica, *Race among Friends: Exploring Race at a Suburban School*

Elzbieta M. Gozdziak, *Trafficked Children and Youth in the United States: Reimagining Survivors*

Pamela Robertson Wojcik, *Fantasies of Neglect: Imagining the Urban Child in American Film and Fiction*

Maria Kromidas, *City Kids: Transforming Racial Baggage*

Ingred A. Nelson, *Why Afterschool Matters*

Jean Marie Hunleth, *Children as Caregivers: The Global Fight against Tuberculosis and HIV in Zambia*

Abby Hardgrove, *Life after Guns: Reciprocity and Respect among Young Men in Liberia*

Michelle J. Bellino, *Youth in Postwar Guatemala: Education and Civic Identity in Transition*

Vera Lopez, *Complicated Lives: Girls, Parents, Drugs, and Juvenile Justice*

Rachel E. Dunifon, *You've Always Been There for Me: Understanding the Lives of Grandchildren Raised by Grandparents*

Cindy Dell Clark, *All Together Now: American Holiday Symbolism among Children and Adults*

Laura Moran, *Belonging and Becoming in a Multicultural World: Refugee Youth and the Pursuit of Identity*

Hannah Dyer, *The Queer Aesthetics of Childhood: Asymmetries of Innocence and the Cultural Politics of Child Development*

Julie Spray, *The Children in Child Health: Negotiating Young Lives and Health in New Zealand*